Praise for
Front of the Class

"Strongly recommended reading . . . *Front of the Class* is the remarkable story of a remarkable man who learned to deal with a marked and all too remarkable affliction."

—*Midwest Book Review, Reviewer's Choice*

"Thank you, Brad, for your determination, your spirit, your compassion, and your perseverance, and thank you for daring to share it with all of us."

—Susan Conners, education specialist,
Tourette Syndrome Association, Inc.

"This book provides a genuine and heartfelt message of hope in the face of a potentially devastating disorder."

—Neal Adams, M.D., MPH, Psychiatric Services,
Journal of the American Psychiatric Association

"Brad Cohen's story is a triumph of hope, determination, will, and relentless good humor. His approach to living with Tourette syndrome proves how much is possible when you expect the best of everyone, especially yourself."

—Peter J. Hollenbeck, Ph.D., professor and associate head of biological sciences, Purdue University

"*Front of the Class* is not just a book about Tourette syndrome. It is a courageous and touching account of one young man's difficulties and triumphs in life."

—Sheryl K. Pruitt, M.Ed., clinical director, Parkaire Consultants and coauthor of *Teaching the Tiger* and *Understanding Tourette Syndrome: A Handbook for Educators*

Front of the Class

How Tourette Syndrome Made Me the Teacher I Never Had

Brad Cohen with Lisa Wysocky

St. Martin's Griffin
New York

www.stmartins.com

Cohen, Brad, 1973–
    Front of the class : how Tourette syndrome made me the teacher I never had / Brad Cohen with Lisa Wysocky. — 1st ed.
        p. cm.
    Includes index.
    "First published in the United States in 2005 by VanderWyk & Burnham."
    ISBN-13: 978-0-312-57139-9
    ISBN-10: 0-312-57139-9
    1. Cohen, Brad, 1973– —Mental health.   2. Tourette syndrome—Patients—Biography.   I. Wysocky, Lisa, 1957– II. Title.
    RC375.C64 2008
    362.196'830092—dc22   2008038734

First published in the United States in 2005 by VanderWyk & Burnham

10 9 8 7 6 5

To everyone who has Tourette syndrome

CONTENTS

FOREWORD

by Jim Eisenreich

I'M JIM EISENREICH and I am a former professional baseball player. Like Brad Cohen, I also have Tourette syndrome, which is a neurological disorder that causes repeated and sometimes debilitating vocal and muscular twitches called *tics*. I first met Brad at a national Tourette syndrome conference when he was in his very early twenties. We were on a young adult panel together and I was awed by his poise, his confidence, and his commitment to education. My impression of Brad, even at that age, was one of a very determined and motivated young man. When you talk to Brad it is very noticeable that he has a frequent vocal tic that can be quite distracting to someone who is listening to him. If I had a vocal tic that severe, I don't know that I could speak in public as much or as eloquently as Brad does. But his vocal tic—or any of his other tics—has never stopped Brad from striving to reach his goals or from educating people about Tourette's.

At that first meeting, Brad and I found we had a lot in common: we both began displaying symptoms at around six or seven years of age; we both were misdiagnosed, had difficulty in school, and were teased mercilessly by other kids. Additionally, we both found something to excel in. For me, it was sports, and a career capped by a World Series win with the Florida Marlins; for Brad, it was his leadership skills and his unique ability to make everyone feel at ease around him. When you listen to Brad talk, you constantly hear strange noises right in the middle of his sentences. But Brad just goes on as if they weren't there, and his ability not to be embarrassed or self-conscious about it makes those listening to him forget about the tics fairly quickly.

Neither Brad nor I know why our brains tell us to do the strange things we do, or why we were chosen to have this disorder. But Brad and I have something else in common. We share a need to educate people about Tourette's and to help others who have the disorder. I have been a spokesperson for the National Tourette Syndrome Association, and in 1996 I began the Jim Eisenreich Foundation for Children with Tourette Syndrome to help children with Tourette's achieve personal success. Brad has become a tremendous teacher of young kids and a wonderful role model. Now, working with coauthor Lisa Wysocky, he has created a book that highlights his amazing story.

Brad's great success in life is based on his unwavering determination to set and accomplish extraordinary goals. He sets his sights very high and doesn't stop until he has accomplished what he has set out to do. Brad Cohen never lets Tourette syndrome prevent him from doing anything he wants to do. We should all think of him when life gets us down.

The beauty of Brad's story is that it is a story for every underdog, for everyone who has ever stumbled in life, for anyone who thinks life has dealt them a little more than they can handle. Brad Cohen is a big inspiration to me and hopefully will be to you as well.

Jim Eisenreich
January 2005

PREFACE

TOURETTE SYNDROME IS A NEUROLOGICAL DISORDER of the brain that causes uncontrollable vocal and muscular tics. Depending on my stress level and a host of other circumstances, I may utter a series of loud "WAH, wah, wah" sounds or an individual "woop" several times a minute. My face may be relatively passive, or parts of my body may be convulsed with what look like spasms. Because I have been twitching and making these loud and uncontrollable sounds, called *barks*, for most of my life, I have had plenty of experience being taunted and even physically attacked. I've also been kicked out of classrooms by teachers. In the 1980s, as I was growing up with Tourette's, doctors knew little about the neurological disorder and the public was barely aware it existed. As a child I even heard adults openly speculate as to whether my behavior meant that I was possessed by the devil. Today people routinely stare at me in the mall, going to a movie or concert is virtually impossible, and dating is a whole other story in itself. I am one of over a hundred thousand people in the United States who have full-blown Tourette syndrome.

If you can imagine a life like this, imagine the difficulty in not only getting a job but excelling in a job that puts you in front of a room full of people. Because I did not get the support and understanding of my peers and teachers growing up, you might predict that would make me think about a quiet job I could do at home—away from rude stares. The lack of support, however, fueled my desire to become the positive and accepting teacher I never had. Of course, the world frequently does not share our dreams; the first twenty-four principals who interviewed me weren't willing to hire someone with Tourette syndrome.

In fact, I have learned that Tourette's is not always a hindrance; the coping skills Tourette syndrome forced me to learn have also given me the confidence to make my dream of being an effective and compassionate teacher a reality. Because of my years of Tourette-based isolation as a child, I believe that staying relentlessly involved in a child's day-to-day well-being is the greatest skill a teacher can bring to the classroom. Today, I tell my students that Tourette syndrome is my constant companion and that without it I just wouldn't be me. Has it been a struggle? Of course. Has it been rewarding? Absolutely.

I think of it this way: we all have a choice between looking at our own cup of life as being half full or half empty. Early on, I chose to view my cup as if it were filled to the brim. Every one of us has some sort of disability. Some disabilities, like mine, are more visible to the outside world. Other disabilities, such as a fear of heights, a lack of confidence, or not being a great reader, are harder for people to see. Whatever your situation, I hope my story is an inspiration to you. I hope it makes you realize that no matter what problems or disabilities you have, you too can make your dreams come true.

In conclusion, I'm here to make a difference. I hope everyone shares my vision of making the world a better place, one step at a time. Education is imperative and ignorance isn't bliss. Please help me pass my message along for those who don't have a voice.

Cheers,
Brad Cohen
January 2005

Acknowledgments

Brad Cohen

I want to acknowledge everyone who has Tourette syndrome. We are our own fraternity and it's great to know there is so much support. I hope this book helps you cope with TS down the road.

How do I say thank you to the many who have helped me get to this point and who have inspired me? First, I need to recognize my immediate family and thank them for their unconditional support. We have been through some tough times, but we always rebound stronger than before. Jeff, Mom, Dad, and Diane, thank you for being there, even when I didn't think I needed you. It's great to know I always had the support I needed. Second, thanks to my extended family for sticking through the tough times in order to celebrate the happy times now. Family is important, and I have learned that I can count on mine.

Thank you to my loyal friends; you mean a lot. I don't take friendships for granted, and you all motivated me to be successful. I wish I could name everyone, but that would be another book.

Thanks to my favorite elementary school in the world, Mountain View. To Jim Ovbey and Hilarie Straka, a special thank you for giving me my dream of being a teacher and allowing me a chance to be in "front of the class." Thanks to all the teachers, especially my second grade team, and my other special friends. Thanks, too, to Stripling Elementary for all your support!

Also, I can't forget the wonderful students I've had the privilege to teach. You are the foundation of the classroom and you helped me be the best teacher I could be. You believed in me when it counted most. I want you to know that I love teaching and I hope you left my classroom an even better person than when you arrived.

Thanks to the following individuals, who have gone out of their way to see this book in print: Sharlene Martin, my agent at Martin Literary Management; Anthony Flacco; Patti Ghezzi, who helped me get started and came up with the great title; Lisa Wysocky for helping me write the book; Corey Gers for the website; and Jim Eisenreich for writing the foreword. Thanks to Andy Lipman, Wendy Bain, Anne Newhouse, and Michael DeFillippo for their guidance; to Jonathon Lyons for his generosity; and, of course, to Meredith Rutter at VanderWyk and Burnham—thanks for publishing me.

Thanks to my fraternity, Alpha Epsilon Pi (AEPi), for believing in me and allowing me to be active, and to the B'nai B'rith Youth Organization (BBYO) for not being my life but giving me a life.

To all my friends at Cobb County's Relay for Life, who help put on one of the best fundraisers in the nation, thanks for allowing me to be your leader. And to the Atlanta Braves and Kory Burke, thank you for allowing me to fulfill my dream of being the Braves mascot. I wouldn't trade that for anything.

I am truly honored that Hallmark Hall of Fame thought so highly of my life story to want to do a movie about me. I'm so grateful to have the chance to share my story with the world. Thanks for believing in me.

Thanks to the Tourette Syndrome Association of Georgia and the National Tourette Syndrome Association. It's been a pleasure working with all of you! I hope my message makes our lives and the lives of future Touretters better down the road.

Lastly, thanks to everyone who has allowed me to be me.

Lisa Wysocky

I want to thank Sharlene Martin, Anthony Flacco, and Meredith Rutter, who all believed in the power of Brad's story, and without whom this account would never have been told. Thanks to Brad's many friends and family members who so generously contributed their time and stories; I just wish we could have used them all. And deep appreciation to Brad Cohen, who invited me into his life and who is a fabulous writing partner and an all-around great guy.

Front of
the Class

1

A "PLAYABLE IDENTITY"

I GREW UP IN ST. LOUIS, Missouri, home of the Arch and home of Cardinals baseball. My parents, Norman and Ellen, divorced very early in my life—so early, in fact, that unlike many children, I was far too young to think that the divorce had anything to do with me. Of course it didn't. By the time I was old enough to even realize that my parents were divorced, that's just the way life was.

To say that I was a very active kid is a complete understatement. At the mall, my younger brother, Jeff, and I were the kids who tore through clothing racks and down the aisles, and generally wore our mother out with our boyhood energy. But the difference between Jeff and me was a question of intensity. Jeff, eighteen months younger, was a typical rambunctious boy—the kind who might be a pain to deal with sometimes, but who was otherwise like most boys.

And me? My energy levels were more manic. My fun seeking was much more frantic than Jeff's, and my excitability level was much higher. By the time I reached second grade, my relentless hyperactivity was understandably a huge concern at home. My mother realized that something was going on and that it was a disturbance deeper and stronger than anything behind Jeff's youthful outbursts.

Back then, Internet access was still a few years away, and there wasn't much information available to answer her questions—or silence her fears. At that time, social resources for conditions like mine were so few and far between that as my symptoms grew deeper, my mother and brother found themselves alone in the house with a virtual stranger. He looked like me, but he was entering all of our lives in staccato bursts of behavior that I couldn't predict, and over which I had very little control. I, like many people with Tourette syndrome, have a short attention span and some mild obsessive behaviors. (Many with Tourette syndrome also have attention deficit disorder, ADD; attention deficit hyperactivity disorder, ADHD; or obsessive-compulsive disorder, OCD.) And so along with the beginnings of facial twitches and rebellious behaviors came the attention span of a gnat.

We all stumbled along, hoping for the best.

My father, who was not a daily presence in our lives, paid just enough attention to my outbursts to dismiss me as an irritating kind of kid. This prevented him from asking himself some hard questions about what was going on. I know my emerging behaviors both embarrassed and disappointed him. I was a subpar version of that idealized firstborn son, the one whose fantasy image lurked in the back of his, and every father's, mind. The irritation that he felt toward me—and that sometimes turned to raging anger—prevented him from having to endure any intimacy with his baffling boy. He could always distance himself by falling back on the familiar pattern of being in a snit over my latest outburst.

Looking back from an adult perspective, I am sure my father also had some feelings of helplessness. Here he was, seeing us only on weekends and trying to establish a new kind of workable relationship with his ex-wife. Some people just ignore what they don't understand and can't fix. Later, I found out that my dad was following advice he had received from several doctors. They told him that my problems were behavioral and that I needed more discipline. I think he has always regretted how he reacted, but, unfortunately, at that point in his life it was the only way my dad knew how to cope.

And this phase was only the lead-in to my problems. The real beginning was at summer camp, before starting the fourth grade. Each year Jeff and I spent at least a month at Camp Sabra, which was about two hours west of St. Louis, near Lake of the Ozarks. I loved it there because I was able to run and jump and swim off a lot of my excess energy without being yelled at. I loved the organized sports, the camaraderie with the other kids, the counselors—everything. But this year, I developed a strange new habit of clearing my throat every few seconds, all day long. Most of the time I had no awareness of doing it.

Naturally, the other kids noticed. But since no one —including my family and me—had ever heard of Tourette syndrome, nothing much was made of my little habit. Mostly the kids thought it was funny, even though as the season wore on, my frequent throat clearing became a near-constant grinding in the back of my throat.

During closing ceremonies at the end of the summer, my counselor gave me an improvised "Froggy Award" for having so amused everyone with my funny noises all season. I wasn't upset by the tongue-in-cheek award or by the hand-lettered paper certificate. Up to that point, my vocal tics had developed only to the extent of throat clearing and an accompanying assortment of odd grunts. I could usually get away with letting people assume I was some upstart kid who made funny little noises as a running joke—and I was happy to let them think so.

Inside, though, my strange behavior was so upsetting and confusing that I did my best not to deal with it at all. So, despite whatever implied mockery may have been behind the Froggy Award, I clearly remember stepping forward to accept it without feeling any awkwardness. In fact, I beamed like any class clown getting reinforcement for his antics. The award and the positive attention helped me to believe—for a little while—that I might be able to bury the weird little behaviors, or hide behind the appearance of an eccentric joker.

Sure, a reputation like that draws a lot of heat from authority figures, but an eccentric joker is an identity you can play when out in the world. People might regard you with annoyance, but they don't feel the need to stare. And when they do look at you, they don't see a freak, they see a playable identity—meaning that, for a little while, I was able to pull it off. Nothing wrong with me, folks—just a funny guy who likes to make funny noises, okay?

In the years since, people have asked if I was hurt by the implied ridicule of receiving such an award. But at that time, a source of wisdom deeper than I could understand was already guiding me to ignore any jabs and to choose instead to accept the element of honor that was there.

I can't take credit for that wise (or lucky) choice, but I've certainly learned how to employ it since. It's amazing to me, whether I'm considering my own life or someone else's, how often I see examples of people reacting with anger or pain to a personal slight without being able to realize that they are in a situation in which they have another choice: they can *decide* that the comment or behavior they consider hurtful might also be legitimately classified as a flattering piece of attention.

No, it won't always work. I just know that my life and my career add up to concrete proof that it often can work. When we decide to experience someone's attention as a positive sign, that can lead to positive outcomes.

With summer over, the dreaded new school year began, with its endless hours of enforced quiet time and its low tolerance for funny, smart-mouthed guys like me who "insist on constantly drawing attention to themselves with subversive little sound effects." That's a direct quote from one of my former teachers.

Have I mentioned how much I hated school? I was not a good student then. I didn't have the attention span to stay quiet very long, so teachers were constantly criticizing me. And, as in the book *Lord of the Flies,* the kids in my school turned on the one child who was different from all the rest. They taunted me, beat me up when they could, and ignored me—when a simple, friendly smile would have gone a very long way.

And these were only the early days of the emerging symptoms. The intruder had been sleeping in the basement of my life, but it was waking up fast. Soon everything was going to be much worse.

On top of my emerging tics, we had recently moved and I was starting a new school, Green Trails Elementary. It was only about eight miles away from our old house, but it meant a new place with new kids and new teachers and no familiarity with anything at all. I was very stressed over both the move and the new school.

To compound these problems, in addition to clearing my throat I had also developed a habit of knocking my knee against the door of the car when I was a passenger. Of course that kind of behavior drove everyone nuts. Who could blame them? And when I insisted, "I can't help it," it's easy to see how people would wonder just what the heck I meant by that. Was I actually claiming that I "couldn't help" being an annoying jerk?

The knee-knocking-in-the-car behavior provoked my father to the point that he would lose his temper and actually hit me to make me stop. The shock of taking a slap, and the fear of getting another, was enough to halt my range of tics for a short while. But the problem was that the tics never stopped for long. Even when I knew I was going to get smacked for it, I found myself repeating the behavior. Remember, Tourette's includes *uncontrollable* neurological behaviors. Telling people with Tourette's to stop a behavior is like ordering someone with allergies not to sneeze.

And so the joker identity quickly became a lot less playable. No one was laughing anymore, particularly after I added yet a third tic to my repertoire, a piercing woop or "bark" that was to become my calling card. Imagine sitting in a classroom next to someone who, several times a minute, emits loud noises such as "RAH . . . rah . . . rah" or "wah . . . WAH." Throw an occasional "WOOP" in there and a continual set of facial spasms, and you are sitting next to me. At times my noises were much louder than they are now, and so during many of my school years I must have been nearly shouting.

The bark appeared to arrive on its own, fully formed as a tic. It seemed to me that one day I wasn't making that sound, and the next day I was. As with my throat clearing, I barked automatically and hardly gave it a thought. It played well enough around the house, but out in public, barking got me noticed. People's amusement quotient isn't at its best when they're confronted with a kid making loud sounds in public. After two or three good yelps in the wrong setting, I found it pretty hard to pass them off as being some sort of goofy sounds that I liked to make just for fun.

Additionally, I was running around like a maniac, so my mother took me to the doctor. He put me on Dexedrine, which was commonly prescribed at that time for ADD and ADHD. I was never diagnosed with ADD or ADHD, but stimulants such as Dexedrine reduced my hyperactivity. Over the next few years, as my behavior progressively worsened, my medication dosages became progressively higher. At the time both my mother and my doctor thought that was the correct treatment for my hyperactivity. Later we would learn it was not necessarily so.

My—and Jeff's—extraordinarily high activity level was one of the reasons for our move to the new house and school. Mom thought we all needed to have a fresh start, so she moved us to a new neighborhood that still had a number of Jewish families and was still reasonably close to a dynamic Jewish Community Center (JCC). My brother, Jeff, loved our new house, our new school, and the new kids to make friends with. Although Jeff is a year and a half younger than I, even at that early stage his greater social ability was a sign of the growing differences between us.

I found the move highly stressful. Adapting to foreign situations had become one of my weakest points. The out-of-control changes inside filled me with a strong distaste for changes elsewhere in my life. Additionally, I kept my fears bottled up inside, which added to my stress and to my tics. I didn't like to share my feelings, and the eventual emotional toll this took was huge. Also, as I wasn't yet able to predict how bad my tics might become in any given situation, going out in public became an increasingly dicey proposition.

With social disaster always lurking outside the door, I craved routine in every other area of my life. The safe predictability of home helped me retain some small feeling of control. But even inside our new home I was not fully comfortable.

For example, my mother's bedroom was on the first floor, while the rooms Jeff and I occupied were upstairs. In our old home, all the bedrooms had been together on the second floor. That difference alone set off my anxiety. I refused to sleep in my room upstairs. Instead, I dragged my pillow and bedspread downstairs and spent every night on the couch in our wood-paneled den, using the glow of the television to ease my fear of the dark. It became important to me to have a night-light of some kind, since darkness promoted uncertainty and uncertainty equaled anxiety. Slowly, my daily and nightly routines became more and more focused on clinging to the familiar and avoiding the unpredictable.

My behavior created a vaguely ominous backdrop. If anyone other than our mother—any child-care professional, for instance—was charged with taking care of us for very long, he or she soon quit. It usually took only a single evening to scare off a baby-sitter. My mother could barely control Jeff's hyperactive behavior, and she accepted the fact that sometimes no one could control mine. My behavior had reached the point that some people, baby-sitters included, found it frightening.

I must admit that at least some of our behavior with the baby-sitters was intentional. Like children being taught by a substitute teacher, we gave our sitters a hard time just because we could. Jeff and I were mischievous boys who enjoyed the chaos we were causing. It was fun to tip over furniture and throw things around the room! But I admit that it often got out of control. Neither of us knew where to draw the line. Our hyper states were fueled by increasing activity, and I can easily see how Jeff and I together were a bit much.

My grandmother Dorothy provided Mom's only respite. She was my mother's mother, recently widowed, and willing to employ her free time in helping Mom out, even on short notice. We called her Dodo, and we adored her. Sometimes Jeff and I spent the night in her little apartment. She was completely accepting of my energy level and my funny noises, even if her downstairs neighbor was not. Every once in a while, he banged on the air-conditioner vent with a broom to get us to quiet down. Regrettably, tics do not care about the time of day or night, or whether the neighbors are angry about the noise.

My childhood was not all doom and gloom, however. A real ray of sunshine came into my life when Mom and Dad chipped in and bought me a terrific green bicycle. I discovered a new source of freedom outdoors—a boy on a bike can speed all over the neighborhood, making all the noises he wants, and no one thinks a thing of it! When I was riding my bike, that terrible, growing conspicuousness that was beginning to dog me everywhere dissolved in the wind and the motion and the exertion of riding.

I named my bike the Green Dragon, and to me its speed was unmatched. I challenged other kids to race, and I usually won. Luckily, the Green Dragon was as resilient as it was fast. It survived two major accidents, one when I propelled it head-on into a brick wall and another when I flipped over a sewage drain and had to be taken to the hospital by ambulance. I got a concussion, but the Green Dragon was unscathed.

The Green Dragon was more than an extension of me. It was a symbol of my physical freedom; it was my disguise. When I was riding the Green Dragon, my condition was invisible. That bike was my most loyal friend—and a real protector. On the Green Dragon, I forgot about my tics and all the problems they were causing for me and my family. Speeding up and down the hills around our neighborhood with the wind in my face, I was like any normal kid. I wished those hills would go on forever.

Since I was in constant motion all day long, Mom signed Jeff and me up for after-school programs at the local JCC. Her thoughts about an active center and organized activities proved to be right. Jeff and I participated in all kinds of sports there, depending on the season: baseball, floor hockey, basketball, soccer. We both loved the place; we could stay all weekend and be thoroughly entertained. I even loved keeping score for the adult intramural basketball games . . . *everyone* yells at ball games.

Optimistic people often tried to reassure Mom that both my brother and I were nothing more than healthy, active boys. And with Jeff, it was true. But it was also true that my behavior was becoming progressively worse, and Mom was having a harder time keeping me in line.

It wasn't just a matter of little behavioral tics that I couldn't suppress; I was having a harder time keeping myself "in line" all the way around. Fear of my mother's displeasure wasn't nearly as bad as the fear that I was losing the ability to control all aspects of my behavior. Whatever the cause, it was becoming extraordinarily difficult for me to get along with other people. Most adults saw me as an overly rebellious, willful kid. But I struggled with the creeping suspicion that my willpower, the basic ability to control myself, was dissolving within me. My behavior had become so bad that it terrified even me.

My poor brother was the one most often in my vicinity, so I frequently picked fights with him. Jeff was more forgiving and understanding than I could expect anyone else to be, but he had his limits, too. Years later, Jeff told me that he often purposely egged me on. He wasn't proud of that fact, as even then he knew I couldn't help my behavior. Some of it, he said, was peer pressure—he was, after all, the brother of the weird kid. But some of it was just the fact that we were brothers and very close in age.

That second fact holds a perverse truth: those fights actually helped me. Much of what I was going through was learning different ways to cope with the strange tics, and the fights helped me in my struggle to appear normal. They shifted attention away from my tics and back onto me. Normal kids get into fights, too.

Mom still hoped most of my tics and hyperactivity would calm down as we continued throughout that school year to settle into our new surroundings. She also thought Jeff and I needed more time with our father. Right after we had moved, he had relocated out of state, and so we now saw him only on holidays and would see him for a longer time in the summer. But Mom's idea about me needing more contact with my father didn't prove to be correct. The tics got worse when he was around.

I now see the increase in my tics, particularly during visits to Dad's place, as being a direct result of the anxiety that was produced by being around a man who did not know how to deal with the rapidly changing behavior of his son. The absence of an accurate diagnosis was causing years of frustration and the development of parenting habits that were counterproductive.

In those days, what my dad was to me was a large male with an unpredictable temperament. In fairness, what a "son figure" I must have presented to him! Each visit was odder than the last. While my tics progressed at a safe distance from him, he only saw the development of my symptoms as if they were stills from a movie. And those scenes weren't long enough to help him find a way to cope.

At least when we were separated by hundreds of miles, Dad could be the fond absentee father. We had great phone conversations every Sunday morning. But on those increasingly rare occasions when I was actually in his presence, he was confronted with a normal-looking boy who possessed some inexplicable need to make himself look and sound ridiculous.

I understood that I was supposed to feel some level of instinctive fondness for my dad and a connection with him as my father, but his positive attention had become virtually impossible to obtain. I always had a guilty sense of relief when it was time to leave his house and go home. But the relief was mixed because I didn't really know if I wanted to go. Sometimes I would cry on the plane on the way home because I was sad to be leaving him, but at the same time it was very nice to get back to my daily routine.

✳   ✳   ✳

At the age of seven, when we were still living in our old house, I had been assigned a "big brother" (in a Jewish mentoring program similar to Big Brothers Big Sisters) and had the great good fortune to be paired with an astoundingly stable, committed volunteer named Steve Mathes. Steve was just twenty-four, and already married and the father of a baby boy, but he still found time to take the big-brother role seriously. We got together every other weekend. We went to Cardinals baseball games, and once we went to see the Harlem Globetrotters. Steve took me to the zoo with his family and had me over for dinner on Friday nights. His wife, Julie, loved to cook and she made solid, basic meals such as meatloaf with pumpkin pie for dessert. It was the kind of comfort food that I wasn't used to at home, as Mom was usually too frazzled by us to cook big meals. Sometimes Steve and Julie invited me to sleep over, and I was always glad to stay. On Saturday mornings, we'd head to the local donut shop. I loved and thrived on the regularity and consistency of my times with Steve. Even after my family moved farther away, Steve and I continued getting together often.

Steve has said that rather than adopting the usual one-on-one role that big-brother programs usually encourage, he instinctively included me as part of his family. Steve somehow knew that the little things, such as watching a grown man shave (as I never had seen my dad doing) were very important to me. He never tried to be a dad, but he helped me see what being a man was all about.

To me, Steve represented all the good in the world because he had very high expectations for everyone, including himself, while at the same time he played fair and behaved like a winner. He saw the best in me when others didn't. As time went on, the unselfish way that Steve and Julie invited me into their family showed me that even though I was different, I could still find acceptance in a normal and safe place. I took great pride in being a part of Steve's family, and we've remained a part of each other's families since then. Steve has been to all my graduations, and his son—who was just one year old when Steve and I first met—is now twenty-three and lives in Atlanta, having attended Emory University. To this day, Steve Mathes remains my strongest male role model.

2

OUT OF CONTROL

ABOUT THE SAME TIME I MET STEVE, when I was in second grade, my hyperactivity and my tics were increasing, so my mother turned to a professional to examine my feelings about the divorce. She dutifully took me to weekly appointments with one psychologist after another. I eventually saw three over the next few years—but I never disclosed much to any of them. To me they were strangers. Their potential to cause trouble for me was unknown, and I had no idea what they intended to do with whatever information they gleaned from me. At that point in my life, I seldom had an encounter with an authority figure of any kind that didn't go badly in one way or another. Regardless of my thoughts on the matter, I now spent an hour each week under interrogation by the enemy, and like a good little prisoner of war, I gave back as little as I could. The scenario usually went like this: they asked a lot of long questions, and I made a lot of short, wary replies. Here's one interaction I remember when I was nine or ten:

"How does it feel when you make a noise or a tic?"

"Relief."

"Do you feel anger toward your mother because your father left town?"

"No!"

"How do you feel when other kids don't want to be around you?"

"Just like anyone would—sad."

"Who do you want to blame when you get in trouble?"

"Myself."

At the time, that was the only answer I could give, because I didn't understand what was happening. Later, after I learned I had Tourette's, I didn't blame anyone, simply because there was no one to blame.

None of the doctors really seemed to need my help or input—even though my parents' divorce had nothing to do with my personality troubles, it got the blame anyway. From my point of view, finding the cause of my condition wasn't nearly as important as finding ways to deal with it—and that was assuming that my emerging jerks and yips and yells could ever be "dealt with" at all.

Soon after I began classes in the fourth grade, at my new school, the subtler effects of Tourette's began. They were little things, mostly, but since I had not yet been diagnosed, they were things we didn't know to expect. Realizing that there were still more unknowns out there that could present themselves was very upsetting. These new little symptoms began appearing like pop-up ghosts in my everyday life, most of all in my struggles with schoolwork. I was too smart to be having so much difficulty.

Although I didn't know it then, while I was at school my mother was engulfed in frantic research, because I had begun doing other things that alarmed her. I was twitching. My face, arms, legs, and neck—major muscle groups twitched without warning and for no apparent reason. Imagine trying to read a book or write out an arithmetic problem when your face and head and neck are regularly twitching so badly that you continually lose your place, whether reading or writing. Every few seconds I'd have to take a moment to reorient myself on the page, then take in as much as I could before the next series of twitches came along. Long passages were a struggle, and every assignment took forever to finish. It really was a very slow process, and I didn't know what to make of it—especially since my cognitive and memory skills were so strong. You see, the actual concepts put to us as students weren't a problem for me, and the logic behind complex ideas was nothing I couldn't handle. The trouble came at the point of contact, the first time my brain took in the information, and I felt it most with anything that involved reading or math.

But my study difficulties paled in comparison to my newest tic—an entirely new era of knee knocking. I mentioned earlier that when I was in the car I'd begun the practice of wobbling my leg back and forth against the door. Now, when I was in the car and sitting next to Jeff, I began swinging my leg just enough to knock my knee against his. Not hard, but just annoying enough to drive any human nuts. The aggravation factor was bad enough, but in this case the worst part was that I honestly had no desire to mess with Jeff or cause trouble. I had no motive for bumping him over and over. But who was going to believe me when my behavior said the opposite? Of course Jeff would demand that I stop, but I couldn't. At that time, I hadn't developed my language skills enough to explain to Jeff that what my body "needed" was the feel of my knee knocking against his knee—in some very specific, certain way. I somehow knew that with the impact would come a feeling that turned off the need. It's hard enough to explain all these years later; I certainly had no capacity for it back then. But I'd guess that the explanation would have sounded too absurd to have done me any good anyway.

You might be asking how this tic went over on visits with my father.

The short answer is that it drove him nuts. The first time Jeff and I got into the car with him and the knee knocking started up, he told me to stop—over and over—and of course I didn't, and before long it wore through his patience like sandpaper rubbing on the skin of an elbow. In his frustration, Dad worked his version of tough love on the situation and popped me across the chin. I began to cry, because I was angry and embarrassed and equally confused. I wanted to stop knocking my knee but I couldn't, so now I was going to have to pay the consequences.

Dad moved me into the front seat. So I went back to knocking my knee against the door. Same thing, looking for that just-right knock. Dad thought I was either mocking him or rebelling by trying to damage his car. Round and round it went.

My mom believed me when I said I couldn't help it. When I got upset, she rubbed my back to calm me down. It helped a lot, but I still didn't talk to her about all the scary things going on in my head. I couldn't tell her how confused I was, or how frustrated. The guilt of adding more to her burden would have been worse than the relief of talking it over with her. By this time I was old enough to realize how much pressure she was under just being a single parent, not to mention being a single parent of two hyperactive kids, one of whom was thought to be a little "strange." So I just kept trying my best to figure it all out on my own. Mom kept hoping I would get used to the new house and the new school and settle down. She was especially worried because my teacher had begun sending notes home about my disruptive behavior.

I should explain that my mom is tall, sunny, and vivacious, with chestnut-colored hair, and she always had a sense of style that her many women friends admired. When Jeff and I were little, Mom sold clothes at a Saks Fifth Avenue department store. After we moved she started her own business selling women's sportswear, often out of the trunk of her car. Women came to our house to try on clothes, and my mother, with a mix of marketing savvy and genuine friendship, turned their visits into real social events. The key to her success was that Mom always gave the impression that she had no worries. It was *her* playable identity.

Mom and the telephone were inseparable, and her favorite place to talk was in our bright kitchen. Her friends often could hear me raising my usual ruckus with Jeff while my mother paced around on the white tile floor. Mostly she talked about frivolous things, but sometimes she and my dad had tense exchanges about child support and whether the check really was in the mail. It often arrived late. But that was—and is—Dad.

My birthday presents, to this day, still arrive late. I decided early on to take the better-late-than-never point of view. Better the check and presents arrive late than not at all. Better Mom and Dad have tense phone conversations than no conversations.

One Sunday, after my usual Sunday morning conversation with Dad, I handed the phone over to Mom. Usually I raced upstairs and found something to get involved in, but this time I stopped halfway up to listen in on the conversation. Mom did all the talking.

I was totally shocked as I listened to her describe my behavior. I seemed to have played a trick on myself by hanging back on the stairs, listening as the raw truth rolled out. Over the phone, Mom recounted one mortifying incident after another. I froze there on the steps. Did I really do all that? My cheeks got hot with embarrassment at the thought of my mother silently observing me while I acted in such strange ways.

I couldn't believe I was that out of control. Mom sometimes had a habit of exaggerating stories; I wondered if maybe that was the case this time. She made the situation sound so bad. When I got back on the phone with my dad, I tried to do damage control and offer assurances that everything was okay. That suited him better. He didn't want to talk about my tics or my poor behavior—he wanted a quick synopsis of the mundane aspects of our lives, such as how I did on my social studies test or how I was doing on my baseball team. I was happy to play along if it got me off the phone without any trouble.

About this same time, Dad took Jeff and me on a special trip to Disney World, where he hoped I would behave more like a typical ten-year-old. I wanted to be a typical kid more than anyone could possibly imagine. I was very excited about the trip, as any kid would be, and I did have a really good time. I loved the ride Space Mountain, and I was enthralled by the Disney characters, especially Goofy, who was my favorite. But in my typically optimistic way, I had envisioned a trip during which Dad and I actually got along—and I am sure he had the same vision. Instead, I wore down his patience with my constant ticcing and hyperactivity, and he got angry. I became discouraged by my father's inability to understand that I could not control my behavior. I hated the fact that I couldn't be what my dad wanted—no matter how hard I tried—and I couldn't wait to go home.

If my father was having trouble accepting me, others in my extended family were even more skeptical. My dad's parents responded to the very mention of my tics with silence. Dad was very much in the bury-it-and-wait-for-it-to-go-away phase that would last until I gained some leadership recognition in my high school years. My cousins were unsure and really didn't want to deal with me if they didn't have to. This all made for some very strained family gatherings. Without Dodo, who regularly came to the rescue and who stood up for Mom, Jeff, and me, I am not sure what kind of relationship I would have with any of my family members today. It made me realize firsthand that approval and acceptance are the only effective weapons against an endless array of cruelties to which anyone struggling with a disability is inevitably exposed. Mom and Dodo gave me those weapons.

✳   ✳   ✳

Nothing changed the fact that my mother was desperately looking for solutions and that I was still out of control. Once, in a grocery store, I actually heard a woman seriously suggest to my mother that I might be "possessed by the devil." It's funny how a remark like that reverberates inside your head long after the moment itself has passed. I know it did terrible things to my already nonexistent self-esteem. What's even worse is that, for a short time, my mother actually seriously considered the concept. Sadly, over time, this particular woman wasn't the only one who suggested that possibility.

None of it mattered to me. I only knew that I continued to struggle at school. Reading an entire chapter in a textbook was like running a race with cinderblocks strapped to my ankles. I knew reading wasn't supposed to feel that way, and I knew that some of the kids who grasped things more slowly than I did nevertheless could read with much more ease. Any reading task, especially assignments of more than a few pages, took a terrible effort. Before starting a new chapter, I'd count the pages to the finish line. Sometimes I'd find that the last page of the chapter wouldn't run the full page, but would contain only a few paragraphs. That made me extraordinarily happy, and reaching that final page was always a treat.

People often ask why Tourette's should make reading such a chore. After all, if I can see clearly, and I can think clearly, and I can handle language, why is it so hard to read? Twitches aside, the best answer I've found so far is to ask a normal reader to imagine trying to read while several people simultaneously snap their fingers in front of your eyes and clap their hands next to your ears. With Tourette's, those forces of distraction exist internally. The outside world sees only the symptoms, when they manifest in the form of twitches and tics. But within the mind of someone with TS, those physical impulses are only part of the picture. The Touretter's attention span is tormented with flashes of broken thoughts and abstract imaginings. They constantly flick and flash like dancing characters filling a screen and blocking the view behind them—and they seem to move entirely of their own volition.

Yes, the tics can sometimes be squelched for very brief periods, but there is a correlative buildup of energy that will eventually force its way out like an explosive sneeze. At that point, the tics are as unstoppable as water spilling over the top of a dam.

I can now see that there was a time—when my tics were emerging—that they and I were both completely out of control. Now, if I have to, I sometimes bite on a pen or chew gum to focus my energy elsewhere. That sometimes temporarily quiets the tics. Various medications have also somewhat softened the decibel level of my woops and barks, but meds also often have debilitating side effects such as drowsiness and weight gain. Over the years I have taken several different medications for my Tourette's, and new drugs are being developed all the time. So, although there currently are no medications that completely stop the tics, there is hope that in the future there will be. But in the fourth grade—for me—all talk of drugs and medication was still very much in the future.

Even though the tics were devastating to me, I never totally despaired. Many with TS are suicidal, but I have never experienced those depths. Maybe there was some gift inside my nature that allowed me to tolerate my high-maintenance constant companion. Although I was distressed by the controversy my behaviors were causing at home and at school, all in all I was curiously upbeat much of the time. Some scrap of identity was left for me by my defining myself as a unique and original person, despite the obvious social stigma. Compared to some of my blander classmates, I never had the problem of walking around feeling unnoticed. I chose to see that as a positive thing.

In that time and place, I could sometimes even fit in as just another kid on the baseball team (where lots of "chatter" is considered a sign of enthusiastic heckling of opponents). And Jeff and I sometimes participated in normal brotherly activities. We used to play baseball with an old tennis ball and use the garage door as a catcher. For a while, I was a Cub Scout and did all the typical Scout activities, including building birdhouses and participating in the annual Pinewood Derby. Jeff and I had hundreds of small toy cars and we spent endless hours in the spare bedroom, which was our playroom, playing with them or our large collection of baseball cards. We often pretended to be baseball players or wrestlers from WWF (now WWE)—specifically Hulk Hogan and Andre the Giant. Those were times when I did many of the things normal little boys do.

But even though I sometimes forgot myself in those brief and blissful moments, the reality was that I was not normal. Rather than shrink from my unusualness, however, I embraced it, deliberately taking on an unconventional appearance that helped add to my exotic quality. I wore my very curly brown hair long and wild, in a white man's version of an Afro. And I dressed in conservative clothes, which made my wild hair stand out all the more. It helped to cultivate a vaguely mischievous persona as well. The image worked, for a while, because my naturally mischievous disposition coupled with my vocal tics projected a picture that made people think I was "up to something"—as if all my little symptoms were part of some secret joke.

I was juggling a lot of eccentricity, but at that point I could still maintain my inner self in familiar situations—and that reinforced my idea that having a specific identity is a basic human need. Anyone can flourish in a given situation, provided the identity they have—or the one they project—allows them to fulfill their daily needs and accomplish a few of their higher ambitions.

I find it interesting that many people in unique situations such as mine have been labeled "unacceptable" by our society. Most people are round pegs and fit in round holes. And that's fine. For them. But those of us who are square or triangular or purple are often looked upon as lesser people. Our media-driven society has made some very shallow citizens out of the round pegs, and there's no better position than that of a classroom teacher for observing the horrible effects that type of thinking is having upon the youngest members of our society. The costs are enormous when our kids give in to the pressure of measuring self-worth in bizarre ways—by wearing the "right" shoes, for example, or having a cool phone. We need to find better ways to educate our children about their, and our, self-worth. Nonmaterial things, such as kindness and loyalty, should count for more than having great hair. As a child, I found that small but regular doses of acceptance and approval continued to power my self-esteem long afterward. In general, for anyone, acceptance and approval together work like some sort of internal fusion reactor, and just run and run and run.

✳   ✳   ✳

When my fourth grade school year finally ended and summer returned, it was time to go back to Camp Sabra. I boarded the Greyhound bus with my pillow in one hand and a backpack stuffed with candy slung over my shoulder. I couldn't wait to see my friends and find out who would be in my cabin. It was going to be so great to get away from the endless reading struggles—and my teacher's scowling face whenever she had to listen to me reading out loud.

I needed the familiarity of summer camp. Since I happened to be good at water skiing, I couldn't wait to do it again—to remember what being good at something actually felt like—and to fit in with the other kids. Water skiing is another of those great sports in which you can yell out anything you want and not get stared at, and, ironically, I usually don't tic when I ski because my concentration is so focused. I do, however, explode later with a barrage of tics that more than make up for the temporary absence of symptoms while skiing.

That summer was truly wonderful—a much-needed and welcome relief. I was very grateful for it, and still am; besides water skiing, summer camp is full of places where a kid with tics can hide. The days whizzed by, and they moved all the faster because I could never shake the apprehension that the next school term was coming and that with it I'd be returning to a place where I could count on my constant companion to keep getting me in trouble. That certainty was a cold cannonball lodged in my stomach. Down deep, I was certain that before long my growing list of symptoms was going to leave me even more of a social outcast than I already was.

Unfortunately, I was right.

3

TICS ARE IN SEASON

AFTER MY GREAT SUMMER AT CAMP SABRA I tried very hard to settle in at school, but it just wasn't happening. No matter what I tried, I was a distraction to everyone, including myself. Now I was in fifth grade, and my noises had gotten much louder. "Woop! Ja, ja . . . JA!" My classmates were beginning to keep their distance, and teachers had absolutely no patience with me.

After one long series of barks, my teacher humiliated me by making me stand in front of my classmates and apologize for making noises. Then she made me promise to stop. I didn't really understand why I needed to do this, but I got up anyway and stood tall in front of the class. I, of course, was not happy about the situation, but then again, I guess my teacher wasn't either. I looked each kid in the eye as I apologized, because I was truly sorry for the noises and the disruptions, even though I couldn't prevent them. And I promised I wouldn't do it anymore, even though I knew it was a promise I could not keep. Of course, as soon as I took my seat I was barking again.

I knew I was making noises; how could I not know? But I didn't know why. So when my teacher challenged me to stand up in front of the class, it changed the way I looked at the noises. If the teacher, someone who is supposed to be a role model, would not accept me, then how could I expect the students to accept me? Her negative attention made me nervous and confused. Classrooms should be safe places for children to learn, but in this class, with this teacher, nothing was safe.

My mother instinctively understood the situation and fought like a tiger on my behalf.

"I was always down at the school, every day," my mom said. "I taught school for five years, so I know what it's like to be a teacher and have a class full of kids. But talking to the teachers and principal about Brad day after day was like beating my head against a brick wall. I might as well have been doing that, for all they listened to me."

As much as the humiliation hurt, that teacher had a huge positive impact on my life. Because of that incident—and many others just like it—I eventually vowed that someday I, too, would become a teacher, but I would be the great teacher I never had. I would be a kind, caring role model for young people and make positive changes in their lives. I knew firsthand how much a few kind words can mean to a child, and how a little positive support can mean the world to a young person. It was a vow that only grew stronger as I grew older.

❈   ❈   ❈

Meanwhile, a friend of my mother's was close enough to the family to notice my problems and to feel personally concerned. One day he checked a thick medical dictionary in search of an explanation for my increasingly strange ways. He found the formal definition of a rare neurological disorder called *Tourette syndrome*, named for Dr. Georges Gilles de la Tourette, a pioneering French neurologist who first described an eighty-six-year-old French noblewoman with the condition in 1885.

Mom took her new-found suspicions to my doctor, who read the definition with great concern and then cried out, "Oh, my God. We made a mistake."

He immediately ordered me off all the stimulants he had previously prescribed to calm my hyperactivity, and then he sent me to a neurologist, who confirmed that I had Tourette syndrome. There we learned that while stimulants can often help with Tourette syndrome, they don't always; at the time, the medical community thought stimulants could make my Tourette symptoms worse. Over the next few months, through her continuing research, my mother became convinced that the Dexedrine I had been taking actually amplified the Tourette's in me and made my condition far more extreme than if the doctor had never prescribed something so strong. Recent medical research, however, does not support that theory.

Over the years I have found that each person has his or her own chemical reaction to medication, and everyone has to find what works for them. My situation with Tourette's and that particular medication was unique to me. Someone else may have had an opposite reaction. While medical studies do not indicate a connection between Dexedrine and my developing Tourette syndrome, my family and I do believe this is how my situation became so severe. Our belief is that my tendency toward TS was an inherited trait, but that the doctor's decision to keep me on the medication, even after the tics began to manifest and after my symptoms continued to worsen, was a choice that actually intensified the disorder's effects. Soon after the diagnosis we switched doctors.

Beyond speculation about what brought TS into my life, there was a large degree of consolation in knowing that my uncontrollable behavior actually had a medical name. Tourette syndrome is rare and certainly strange, but it is still a known and an understood neurological condition in the world of medicine. That was a huge relief, as it is so much easier to deal with a specific problem than an unknown. Plus, I could finally explain my tics—to others and to myself.

Now, at least when I was at home, I didn't have to fear having my unconscious or unstoppable tics interpreted as willful misbehavior, even though I'm not sure my father was fully convinced. I think he suspected at times that I'd just come up with a foolproof excuse to continue being obnoxious and to torment other people.

Of course, that point of view is exactly what makes Tourette's socially dangerous for anyone who suffers from it. Without meaning to, my father taught me my first lesson in coping with the negative reactions that are part of everyday life for people who vocalize in movies, libraries, restaurants, waiting rooms, and elevators—anywhere silence is expected. And funerals? Please.

Now that my mom had an answer to give, she couldn't wait to tell others that there was a real medical condition causing my problems. As for me, I was glad these medical definitions offered explanations for my growing troubles, and I was happy to accept any slack that I might be cut for it. My one small problem was that Mom knew every little bit of information for some time before she chose to share it with me. She first went through a period of figuring things out for herself, then working through them with family and friends, then finally with teachers and with me. I was a little perturbed that I was at the end of the information list, but by the time something trickled down to me, Mom knew just how to explain it so that it made sense. And she always, always kept it as positive as circumstances would allow.

None of the medical literature, however, had anything to say about how I was actually supposed to live with all this stuff. Mom often called members of the Tourette Syndrome Association and fired off endless questions. When she got the answers, she would share them with my teachers, my dad, and my grandmother Dodo. They were all astounded that my odd ways actually had a medical name. To them, it made no sense that there was some sort of recognized medical condition that made a person twitch and make noises. No one had ever heard of such a thing. This was long before Tourette's became a highly rated topic for television dramas. It really struck them as odd—as if they had been told my condition was the result of witchcraft.

By this point, my mother was really having a time of it. She was suffering from extreme guilt, thinking that she should have instinctively known that the medication could have caused some of the problems. She thought that maybe if she had stayed married I wouldn't have had so much stress and anxiety, and then maybe I wouldn't have all these strange tics. Then she thought God was punishing her for some unknown thing she had done. Or not done. She was lonely and fearful and for years lived one day at a time. In addition to all that, Jeff and I literally ran Mom ragged with our hyperactivity, and her emotions were on a constant roller coaster.

My mother also hid her devastation over the knowledge that there is no cure for Tourette's. Each day after school, no matter what grim news about my condition she may have learned, Mom shielded me from her anxiety and remained bubbly and upbeat. She continued to hope that if she had more information and more support it would help my teachers in how they worked with me. She wanted to find strategies for the classroom, so she found a local chapter of the Tourette Syndrome Association and we excitedly planned to go to its next meeting. We can't remember now whether I was in grade five or six at the time, but in any event Mom's thinking was that she could get some ammunition for dealing with the school system. Then, as Jeff and I had never met anyone with TS—other than myself—we could get together with others who had been diagnosed. Maybe some of them could even become role models for me. Or friends. I was having a very lonely time of it.

I know Mom had our best interests at heart, but things didn't go exactly as planned. The meeting was held in a church basement, in a dark, low-ceilinged room that made us feel uncomfortable the moment we walked into it. The members of the support group, mostly adults, were all crowded into this little room. It was an interesting group, as they all had varying degrees of Tourette's that manifested in different ways. There were the eye blinkers and the nose twitchers, the foot stompers and the neck jerkers. Often these symptoms were all seen in the same person. Then there were those who yelped, coughed, grunted, barked, and shouted. Some touched other people obsessively, or repeatedly banged their head on the nearest handy object. And there were a few who had coprolalia, a much rarer symptom of Tourette's that involves shouting obscenities.

The people who had Tourette's all displayed symptoms far worse than mine, and I was disappointed to find that none of the few kids there were enrolled in public school. All had been sent home to be tutored—privately—either at their own request or at the request of school administrators. I tried talking with a man, but he was constantly making loud screeching noises and flinging his arm in my face—never hitting me, but coming within millimeters each time. I kept my head still and tried not to embarrass him, because I knew he couldn't help it. But the first time he did it, I was so startled I jerked backward and almost fell off the folding chair I was sitting on.

The people had several things in common, I discovered. It was quite obvious that none of them were social. No one there was even trying to be accepted in mainstream society. The adults were all unemployed, many were on some sort of disability plan, and the kids with Tourette's were home, not doing much of anything.

The adults in charge were upbeat and optimistic, but the group members shared a prevailing pessimism about how hard it was to cope. This viewpoint was in direct conflict with my positive nature and the positive spin Mom taught us to put on hardships. Where, we wondered, were all the positive people with Tourette's? Where were the people with Tourette's who were trying to live in society, who were persevering day after day to make a better life for themselves and their families? They certainly were not in this room.

My mother had hoped that the people at this support group meeting would show me that I could live a full and normal life. Instead, these people had embraced a life of sadness and despair. Mom, Jeff, and I left the church basement knowing it would be hard to return.

The positive I drew from this meeting was that it allowed me to see the other side of Tourette syndrome. It allowed me to see other people with Tourette's—people with symptoms far worse than mine—and experience the discomfort of being around them. More importantly, the meeting allowed me to see what my existence could become if I let Tourette's take over my life. The people I met that day were so down and depressed that I made a conscious decision not to be like that. I didn't want to be someone who didn't participate in life and who then complained about it. I wasn't going to let Tourette's dictate who I was as a person. I wanted to be seen as "Brad, the funny guy, and oh, yeah, he has Tourette's," not "Brad with Tourette's, and oh, by the way, he's kind of funny."

I also didn't want my mom to be depressed. I saw how easily a negative attitude could infect the people in my home and pull us all down. So in several ways, this dark, disheartening meeting became another pivotal experience in my life.

One example of my decision to take a positive approach is my viewpoint about attending movies. With TS it is very difficult for me to go to a movie because my barking noises distract other people who, like me, have paid their hard-earned money to watch the movie. But rather than despair about the fact that I can't go to the movies, I look at it from a different angle. I think of it as choosing not to go. Certainly I can go if I really want to. The Americans with Disabilities Act (ADA) has ensured my right to attend public events such as movie showings. Instead of going on a Friday night and disrupting the movie with my series of woops and rah-rahs, if I really want to see a movie I go late on a Sunday morning or at another off-peak time when there won't be a lot of people there.

Another way of looking at it is that I have a very wide circle of friends and my social life is quite full. I always have something to do, so if I have to wait until a movie comes out on video or DVD, or until it is shown on television, that's okay. But to get dejected about the fact that I "can't" see a movie is counterproductive, because if I really want to, there are ways to do it.

The support group meeting, in a roundabout way, also reinforced my never-say-never philosophy, especially as it relates to Tourette's. That day, I learned that I didn't want Tourette's to hold me back from anything in life that I chose to experience. Since then, I have realized that a positive outlook breeds success, just as a negative outlook breeds failure. How can you not have some success when you make a point to surround yourself with positive and successful people? It is virtually impossible. Besides, people don't want to hear all your complaints. If you ask others how they are doing, do you really want to hear how sad and depressed they are? Of course not. So I have made it a point always to be positive, even if I am having a very tough day.

What the support group meeting did not do was give me ideas for how to cope with the members of my extended family. They turned out to be just as skeptical about Tourette's as my teachers were. My relatives just couldn't believe I had no control over the strange noises and twitches and compulsive knee knocking. It was easy for me to see that my father, my grandparents, and my aunts, uncles, and cousins were all uncomfortable around me. You know things have changed when all of a sudden your grandparents don't want to take you out to eat anymore because you embarrass them. These were my dad's parents, and they thought I was just a troublemaker who wanted to be the center of attention.

My uncle Stu, who is my dad's brother, said he didn't think his parents ever really understood Tourette's.

"Brad's grandfather I think was more tolerant about it than his Nana was," Stu recalled. "She would visibly cringe every time Brad made a noise. Every time. I can't imagine how terrible that must have made Brad feel. She never understood the concept of Tourette's or that Brad really had no control over his behavior. I think at the time she felt that she was being punished, and she worried about that. She did love Brad, but she was a worrier."

My wild behavior only encouraged the worrying. In addition to the barks and woops, I developed some additional strange tics during the course of grades five and six. Off and on I had a smelling tic—a strong urge to sniff things, especially books and paper. Newspapers were the worst. Every time I saw a newspaper, I'd have to smell every section of it. After ten minutes of smelling the newspaper, my nose was black from the ink.

I tried to stay away from newspapers, but then I started smelling the pages in my schoolbooks. Imagine sitting in class next to a kid who every few minutes popped his head down to the floor, took a big whiff of his books, then popped back up again.

I also began chomping my teeth so badly that I once chipped a tooth while drinking out of a glass cup. In order to help counteract this tic, we bought a mouthpiece similar to those worn by football players. I hoped it would help, but it just made things worse, as all I thought about after that was chomping my teeth. The urge to do it over and over again was irresistible. (Now, as an adult, I should still use a mouthpiece at night, but I chomp down so hard on them that I keep breaking them, so I'm trying to do without.)

With Tourette's, tics often come and go. After the chomping tic left, the touching tic began. Not only did I need to touch things, I needed to touch them in a certain way. Sometimes I needed to touch something with my left hand, then my right, then my left again, alternating hands until I touched the object just perfectly. That tic gave way to the sound tic. When turning up the volume on the TV, I needed to do it in a particular way. The volume had to be just so. The same was true with the radio in the car, and the slamming of the car door, and the hanging up of the telephone. If things didn't sound just right, I'd do whatever it was over and over and over again until it made that perfect sound, the one I needed to hear. Even though I was never diagnosed with obsessive-compulsive disorder, this is very typical of OCD behavior.

So you can see why my extended family thought I was a bit odd. And it didn't help that Jeff was also hyperactive. It got to the point that my aunts and cousins didn't want to be around us, the "wild kids," and our already strained family gatherings became less frequent.

✳   ✳   ✳

During all this, Mom did her best to keep both Jeff and me active. I tried my hand at music, playing for a time both cello and trumpet. I wasn't good, but it was fun, and the tics weren't so bad when I was playing. It also got me out of the dreaded classroom—anything to get me out of class.

But sports were my salvation. I enjoyed playing three positions on a local baseball team: catcher, second base, and outfield. I also played soccer, swam, took karate, and rode my bike. I loved the physical activity, even though I never excelled at any one sport. Who ever said you had to be good at something in order to enjoy it?

The other positive effect of sports was that I was put in contact with other kids. My circle of friends had shrunk fast, as I changed from being the funny kid with the froggy voice to the weirdo who made all those noises. Additionally, new medication I was taking for my TS was causing me to gain weight—thirty pounds in just a few months. So, in addition to being a weirdo, I was becoming the fat kid on the block. Let's see. I was now the strange fat kid who made noises and had no friends. How's that for a challenge to your self-esteem?

Most of my "friends" by this time were Jeff's friends. He'd invite them over to the house and I'd end up playing with them, as we were so close in age, and really, how else was I going to spend my time? Sometimes we'd play "home run derby" and try to hit the ball over the neighbor's house. One time I actually succeeded! But I didn't want to always hang with Jeff and his friends. Even at that age I realized that even though Jeff didn't mind sharing, he needed his own time with his own friends.

"Because Brad really didn't have any friends at all, I was probably the one who spent the most time with him," agreed Jeff. "I stood up for him over and over, time after time, but kids are mean and most of them didn't listen. A lot of them were pretty cruel to Brad."

Sports inevitably provided the social interaction I needed. As I became part of a team—whether in the outfield or on second base, sitting in the dugout, or even in the water when I swam—I could make all the noises I wanted and it wasn't really a big deal. Running down a soccer field with a group of screaming kids gave me the same privilege. I was with other boys my age and we were having fun and working toward a common goal. We did team things together and lived shared experiences. Only in sports could I have this kind of normal, everyday life. I loved every minute of it.

In hindsight, it was good that I had found a home of sorts in sports, because my social life was about to reach a new dimension of hell. I was getting ready to start junior high.

4

The Wonder-Bread-and-Miracle-Whip Diet

I HAD HIGH HOPES for junior high. I knew it was going to be a challenge because it brought several elementary schools together and so there would be a lot of new kids to meet, but I viewed that as a great opportunity to make friends. Not new friends, because at that point I didn't really have any friends, but with new kids around maybe someone would be able to look past my tics and like me just for being me.

My hopes were not to be fulfilled. I ended up a loner, constantly mocked, desperately praying I wouldn't get beaten up when I stepped off the school bus. I gave a big sigh of relief each day when I finally got home where I was safe with my mother and Jeff.

Jeff was the one person besides my mom who was never embarrassed by my tics. "I always knew Brad couldn't help it. I never hesitated to go places with Brad, but I was always observant of how everyone else looked at him," said Jeff. "Sometimes I looked right back at people who were staring and tried to get them to think it was me making all the noises. At home we fought a lot and I teased him sometimes, but now I think that was more because we were eighteen months apart in age than because of the Tourette's. We fought, but we always supported each other."

My weight was still a problem, and I constantly drank soda. In fact, I drank so much Coca-Cola growing up that if the restaurant didn't offer free refills, our tab was very high. Because McDonald's and other fast food places near us didn't offer free refills, when we went out we often went to Friday's restaurant, where refills were on the house.

Although I regularly chugged soft drinks, my absolute favorite comfort food was a Wonder-Bread-and-Miracle-Whip sandwich—not exactly a healthy snack, but one I constantly craved during school and frequently ate after school. Eating one was a sign that I was home and had safely survived yet another day of junior high.

Eating may have been one of my favorite times at home, but at school it was one of my worst times. Inside the junior high cafeteria, I sat in my baggy jeans and long-sleeved flannel shirt at a table by myself—no one wanted to sit with the kid who barked. Almost daily, as soon as no teachers were watching, a group of kids would come by and mock me by making the same noise or tic I was making at the time. Talk about feeling uncomfortable! And it just got worse and worse, because as my stress level increased, so did the number and volume of my tics. "Woop, woop . . . FA, fa, FA!"

Kids routinely danced circles around me while I tried to eat. They imitated the noises I made and laughed at their own impersonations, while I stared into a tray of tasteless cafeteria food. I tried to ignore them and eat my lunch, but that was impossible. I was a sitting duck. Sometimes I tried to explain that I had Tourette syndrome, but they never listened.

I guess it made them feel better to put someone else down. But it just made me want to go home. It also made me want to throw my food at them. I wanted to yell and scream in frustration and beat the tar out of them. But I didn't. I didn't do any of that because I knew it would just make it harder for me if I did. Instead, I went to the nurse's office.

By this time I was on Haldol, a medication I took for TS that caused both fatigue and an increase in appetite. At school, I had to go to the nurse's office to get my meds, and over time the nurse and I struck up a friendship of sorts. Her office window looked out into the cafeteria, so she could see that I was having a bit of trouble. One day she invited me into her office to eat lunch. I can't tell you how grateful I was for this unexpected respite. One day turned into another, and then another. Pretty soon eating in the nurse's office became a lunchtime habit and a much-needed break from the mockery and taunts of the other students.

The school bus was another difficult place. Mom often drove us to school, but just as often I rode the bus. Kids, particularly the older ones, routinely gave me a hard time about the noises I made. One day a boy who was a year ahead of me got several of the other kids to join him in his taunts. I tried to stick up for myself, but that only fueled their fire. That afternoon the kid made it a point to sit directly in front of me and continue his harassment. He quickly began mocking me and slapping me on my head, and before I knew it other kids had joined in. The bus driver should have seen us by this point, but he was oblivious. As the swings came—each harder and faster than the last—I tried to defend myself. Finally, the bus driver saw us, broke up the scuffle, and pulled us off the bus. We hadn't yet left the school parking lot.

The kid who initiated the fight and I both ended up in the principal's office. When I learned that we would both be put into in-school suspension, I couldn't believe it. I was being punished for being attacked for something I couldn't control. In-school suspension meant sitting in a little room with four white walls with nothing on them. Lunch was brought to you and no noises of any kind were allowed. I did my best to observe the no-noise rule, but my best effort was a miserable failure. Obviously, after a day of this my tics were as bad as they had ever been. When I got home and Mom saw the state I was in, she called the principal and gave him a piece of her mind. It wasn't pretty, but she made sure I would never get put into in-school suspension again.

That was the first chink in the school's armor, giving a positive aspect to that awful ordeal. My mother continued to lobby with ceaseless resolve to remedy one injustice after another, as I was continually being punished for having Tourette's. Initially she didn't have much luck, but over time the staff began to listen to her.

My math teacher at the time, a tall, skinny man who towered over his students, was particularly difficult. He was a stern man who seldom smiled, and he had no tolerance for my tics. He thought I was doing "the hiccups" on purpose; he truly believed I could control them and that I was only ticcing to get attention. Not too far into the school year, he began putting me in time-out whenever my tics started to bother him, which was pretty much constantly. He started sending me to time-out several times a week. I began having trouble concentrating in class because I was trying so hard not to tic.

Time-out at this school meant being sent to another math teacher's class and sitting quietly in the corner facing a wall until the period ended. I hated this and also thought it was a stupid idea. Because of tics beyond my control, I had already disrupted one class. Now I was in another teacher's classroom interrupting her class with my noises. I was the perpetual "kid in the corner." The teacher knew I had been sent to her class because I had already disrupted my own class, so she automatically treated me as a "bad" kid without knowing all the circumstances. So, for many math classes, I sat in the back of a strange classroom, staring at another plain white wall, trying desperately to be quiet, and rarely succeeding. I was embarrassed, but there wasn't much I could do. If I turned around, the teacher got mad. I did try to listen, though, and I must have picked up some of the concepts because I passed the class. And that's how in the seventh grade I literally learned math . . . backward.

From that point on, my mom insisted that she and I have a say in what teachers I would have. She made sure they were educated about Tourette syndrome, and if someone couldn't (or wouldn't) teach me, she made sure the principal found a teacher who could. As a family, we discussed switching to a private school, but I didn't want that. I didn't want to be treated differently because I had Tourette's. My parents always thought I wanted to stay in public school because it offered Spanish and the private school near us didn't, but that wasn't the case. I wanted to take Spanish, but much more than that, I didn't want to use Tourette's as an excuse. I wanted to be normal, and I wanted friends. I knew I just had to work harder at both.

*　*　*

When I turned thirteen, it was time for me to celebrate my Bar Mitzvah, the Jewish ceremony of passage into manhood. Jewish girls have their own Bat Mitzvah ceremony at the same age. Having a Bar Mitzvah is one of the most significant events in the life of a Jewish boy, and it is an amazing thing to witness. Basically, the Bar Mitzvah is a ninety-minute religious service led by a thirteen-year-old in both English and Hebrew. That's a lot of pressure for any kid, and an almost impossible task for someone with Tourette's.

I, like most Jewish boys, began Hebrew school in the fourth grade and prepared myself for several intense years of study. (This was in addition to the regular public school that I attended.) Even though I was having problems in school, there was never any doubt in my mind that I would have a Bar Mitzvah. It was a given. Many people in my extended family didn't think I would ever be able to get through the ceremony because of all the pressure it puts on young men—stress and anxiety are known to increase the symptoms of Tourette's—but my mom never thought twice about it. She knew I would do well. It would be my day to shine.

But I had a few years of Hebrew school to get through first. Mom and I realized early on that I would need a special tutor to work with me, and the one-on-one help ended up play-ing a big part in my Bar Mitzvah success. Still, although I thrived in the tutor-pupil setting, I wasn't quite so triumphant in the religious classroom. Specifically, my barking was getting me in trouble again. No matter how hard I tried, I could not suppress my tics enough to please my Sunday school teachers. When it got to the point that I knew I could never please them, I gave up trying and started acting silly in class on purpose. What did it matter? One way or another I was going to get in trouble, and this way at least I got some positive attention, if only from my classmates. So I would wisecrack and carry out all the outrageous dares that others challenged me to do. Of course, before I could go too far, I was on my way to the administrator's office, snickering and dancing all the way. Now, no one likes to be sent to the administrator's office during Sunday school —except me. To me it was well worth it because for one brief moment I had everyone in the Hebrew class on my side. I felt that we students were all one against the teacher. I was part of a group and they liked me, if only for the silly things I was doing to make the teacher mad. If my memory serves me correctly, one day I even set a personal record for the number of times I was sent out of the room.

Despite the tics—and the time spent in the administrator's office—I learned all I needed to learn, and before I knew it, my Bar Mitzvah was just days away. When it came time for the cer-emony, my family—except for my mom and Jeff—were all on edge about my propensity for unpredictable and bizarre behav-ior. The thought of my odd ways being showcased for all to see filled them with dread.

Mom and Dad felt strongly, however, that I should have this rite of passage. They had put their differences aside and joined forces to stage a typical over-the-top Bar Mitzvah in my honor. Most kids my age were invited to the Bar Mitzvahs of many of their classmates, their friends from the neighborhood, and distant cousins they rarely saw. I didn't get many invitations. But that didn't stop Mom from inviting "everyone and their brother." Surprisingly, most of the adults showed up.

This was also one of the few times since the divorce that both sides of my family were all together. I have to say that Mom and Dad did a great job of keeping Jeff and me out of their problems and out of the divorce. They both worked hard to be cordial when they were in each other's company, and the rest of the family followed suit. Together, Mom and Dad gave me my Bar Mitzvah party; it was my day and everyone recognized that.

Looking back, I realize that I probably should have been scared to death. Some of my distant relatives hadn't seen me in three or four years, and they remembered me as that cute little kid with the big Afro. I still had the Afro, but this would be the first time they would see me with Tourette's, and I wanted to be sure they saw me as a man, not as a strange kid who continually made faces and "burped." The grown-up image I wanted to convey was tough to devise as I, in many ways, was still quite immature. I was still the joker, and much of my humor was only funny to other immature kids. I was visibly self-conscious around others, with good reason, and dialogue with someone outside my immediate circle was often painful for both parties. But because I had to deal twenty-four hours a day with my bizarre tics and the often negative response others had to them, I was far more mature in other ways than most kids my age.

Much of my family's fear and the actual reality of my Bar Mitzvah revolved around the fact that people still did not understand Tourette's. In 1986, the year of my Bar Mitzvah, Tourette's wasn't seen as commonly as it is now. Whether that's because most people with Tourette's were like the people we saw in the support group and stayed home all the time, or there just weren't as many cases, I really don't know. I do know that there are several hundred thousand people in the United States with Tourette's, if you include people with milder forms of the disorder who remain undiagnosed.

But these numbers were far from my mind during my Bar Mitzvah. It was my big day and I was pretty excited. Was I making noises? Sure. Was I twitching? Of course. But I had control—of myself and of the ceremony. I went up to the bema (the raised enclosure around the altar) and read both English and Hebrew very successfully. I more than showed all the doubters that I could do it, and do it well.

Doing well was especially important to me because my tics were really bad around the time of my Bar Mitzvah, with lots of head jerking, shoulder shrugging, and rapid eye blinking. I was ticcing so frequently that sometimes I was unable to concentrate on the conversations I was having. I would lose my train of thought, and I couldn't stay still as my shoulders shrugged back and forth with rapid movement. Oh, and be sure to add my barking noises to all that.

I'm sure some of the tics were the result of so many people thinking I wasn't going to be able to pull this off. I badly wanted to prove them wrong, and in fact, I did prove them wrong. While speaking, I was concentrating so hard on the ceremony that I didn't really tic much. This is a normal thing for me. When I concentrate really hard on doing something, such as giving a speech or talking, I don't tic as much—everything seems to disappear into calmness like snow melting on a warm winter afternoon. I made up for it later, of course, letting out a massive load of twitches and odd noises. But by then the pressure was off. I had proven my point.

It was a very positive ceremony for me in many ways. First—in my faith if not by law—I was now a man. That was a huge milestone. But more importantly it was a turning point with at least some of my family, and others close to my family, because they finally saw me as more than my tics. They saw me get through this very intricate ceremony, and they realized that behind the funny mannerisms I had at least some intelligence. For the first time they had to pay attention to me for a prolonged period of time rather than ignore me or turn away, and they saw what I dealt with on a daily basis. At that point, some of them finally got it. Some of them finally realized that I could not control my twitches and tics. They finally understood Tourette's.

After the ceremony we all went to a big hotel for a luncheon in my honor. Mom and Dad had gone all out and arranged for a dance floor, a band, a caricature artist, and a photographer. Of course, the whole thing was caught on video. Initially, I was a little disappointed that I didn't have any friends to share the event with, but I didn't let that ruin my day or stop me from having a good time.

Having the support of at least a few people besides Mom and Jeff was a huge deal to me. It was validation, friendship, and relief all rolled into one. With all that came my full understanding of how much harder I had had to work to be here on this day than other kids my age. I could have been bitter, but instead I was proud. Even though school—and life—often got the better of me, there was never anything I thought I couldn't do because of Tourette's. I could do whatever I wanted to do; I just had to suck it up and find a way to make it work. If it meant spending more time than a "normal" person would to read a certain number of pages, then I had to spend the time and do it. And I did. If that meant I had less time to watch TV or do something else I enjoyed, then that's just how it was. I had Tourette's and I had to make sacrifices sometimes. I learned to make the best of it and get on with things.

In school, I never liked it when my teachers treated me differently because I had Tourette's. I wanted to be treated just like everyone else, so I made sure that I had my homework done every day, no matter how much effort it took.

Although TS made school difficult enough, the really hard part about school was my lack of friends, and sometimes I would get upset about that. But as I got older I kept one thought in mind: did I really want to be friends with people who made fun of me? Of course not. So I was patient and waited for people to look beyond the Tourette's and realize that I had many good qualities. And finally it happened. It started with my Bar Mitzvah and the people there who learned to look past the tics and twitches. Once they did, they finally saw Brad, and they found that they liked him. People began to accept me for who I was as a whole person. That attitude spread to a few people at school and at the JCC, and before I knew it life was a little bit easier.

After the Bar Mitzvah, I also became friends with some of the older people in my neighborhood, and through them my social skills began to improve. I often asked to help with their yard work, shovel their snow, or baby-sit, and I gained a great deal of confidence in a job well done.

My big brother, Steve Mathes, also saw the positive after-effects of my Bar Mitzvah. He observed, "Having a Bar Mitzvah is an incredible accomplishment, especially for someone like Brad who had to work ten times as hard as most kids. Brad was a lot more confident afterward, and I think people saw that confidence and treated him more respectfully because of it."

My Bar Mitzvah had truly opened many doors for me, but there was one door that still hadn't opened. I was determined to conquer my problems at school.

5

INTRODUCING THE STRANGER

DURING MY JUNIOR HIGH YEARS, my mother was now finding lots of information on Tourette syndrome from several different sources. She was in regular contact with the Tourette Syndrome Association and also made use of the library at Washington University, which was right in St. Louis. While the information was interesting—and helpful—it wasn't all that positive. There was no hope of a cure.

One morning when I was still thirteen, a representative from the Tourette Syndrome Association called my mom with some pretty good news. The *Sally Jesse Raphael Show* was filmed in St. Louis, and its producers had agreed to devote an entire show to Tourette syndrome—something that to our knowledge had never been done before on network television. The best part was that I was invited to be on the panel!

It all came about at the last minute, so I didn't really have time to get nervous. Mom came to school and pulled me out of class and told me I was going to be on television. That was pretty cool, but I was more excited about getting out of school for the day than about being on television. I was excited about anything that got me away from the constant harassment and the stress of the classroom. We didn't have time for me to go home and change, so I showed up at the studio in my usual baggy jeans and untucked flannel shirt. Upon arrival, we were escorted to the show's waiting room, in TV lingo called the *green room*, where we joined other people who were going to be on the show—a doctor and several high school kids with Tourette's. It was an interesting group, as it always is when you get a roomful of Touretters together.

Of our little group, I was the most vocal with my tics—so vocal, in fact, that the producers were nervous that I would distract from the discussion panel, and they ended up pulling me from that part of the show. I can't tell you the disappointment I felt. It was like being rejected from a group of rejects, and, at the time, I was really hurt. If the producers really wanted to show what Tourette's was like, they should have embraced the fact that I was there. The goal of the show was to educate people about Tourette syndrome. For the purpose of displaying Tourette's in both an audio and a visual setting, I should have been their perfect guest.

Just before the show started, the producers brought Mom out to sit in the audience. I ended up staying in the green room during most of the show. Then, during the final segment, they sat me in the audience with Mom long enough to chat with Sally. I was surprised at how much of the show was plotted, with the producers and Sally going over and over the questions with the guests and helping them frame their answers in sound bites rather than in paragraphs. I know that makes for good television, but it rattled me at the time. I was already confused and disappointed by not being able to take part in the discussion onstage, and now I had to remember to talk a certain way.

When Sally came into the audience to talk to me, I was very tense. My tics were both audible and visible, which was good for the viewing audience, but I was trying hard not to let the tics distract me to the point that I couldn't answer her questions correctly. And then the first question she asked was not the first question we had rehearsed. That threw me off. As a result, my answers were short almost to the point of being monosyllabic. Sally asked routine things, such as when was I diagnosed and what was it like to have TS. I was nervous, but I think I did okay. I can now watch the video of that show and see a plump, uncertain young boy with an Afro who was visibly struggling, but who did indeed turn out to be the ideal guest. I looked and sounded like a typical person with Tourette syndrome. Perfect.

A lot of positives came out of my appearance. The experience made me see firsthand how even among compassionate people—such as the producers and the members of the audience—tics are often at complete odds with other people's needs and circumstances. It wasn't my fault that I had TS, but I had to be aware that there were some instances in life in which I had to go around the brick wall rather than plow straight through it. I couldn't be onstage, but I was a part of the show and I had been given a chance to make a difference. In hindsight, it doesn't matter whether I was onstage or not; it matters that I was there and that my presence helped people gain knowledge of Tourette's. That was a good learning experience for me, and one I have recalled time and time again in my daily life. I do not let

Tourette's limit my experiences, but how I enjoy those experiences might be different from how they are enjoyed by a person who does not have TS. Not better, not worse, just different.

By the time the show finished taping, the people in the audience were really in my corner. They were supportive. It was then that I first realized that a little bit of education about TS—or anything, for that matter—could go a long way. On the way out of the studio, everyone treated me like a star. Everyone wanted to talk to my mom and to me, and well-wishers surrounded us. That was a strange feeling, as it was the first time I had received any positive attention for having Tourette's. It certainly beat having lunch alone.

Before the show aired, my mom called all our relatives, and for a short time I was a celebrity in our family, too. The fact that a nationally televised program would devote an entire show to Tourette syndrome and include me in that show was not lost on my family members. It was another tiny drop in that little bucket of validation, and a few more of my relatives began to come around in their ideas about me and about Tourette's.

The show also made great strides in creating public awareness of Tourette syndrome on a national level, and I applaud Sally Jesse Raphael and her producers for doing such groundbreaking television. It was a bit disorienting for one young teen with Tourette's—me—but I am very glad to have played a part in building some initial consciousness of TS nationwide.

✳   ✳   ✳

As most of my classmates were in school when the *Sally Jesse Raphael Show* aired, they didn't see it and didn't get to realize what a star I now was—me along with the eight thousand other people who were on television that day! But Mom made the teachers at school aware of the program, in addition to continuing to pester anyone who would listen, telling them about the hard time I was going through.

Mom had been working hard to educate the teachers, but what about my fellow students? Who was going to educate them? My principal, an innovative guy named Bill Myer, listened to my mom, and he had an idea. By this time I was fourteen and in eighth grade. It was spring, and there was an orchestra concert during school that the entire junior high was attending. I was sitting in the back of the auditorium, making my noises as I always do. Maybe this day was a little worse than usual, because I knew at some point Mr. Myer was going to mention Tourette's.

Sure enough, after the concert, Mr. Myer got up on the stage. He was a dark-haired, well-dressed man in his middle years who was well liked by both teachers and students. He respected others, and they in turn respected him. With everyone's full attention directed toward him, he asked, "Did you hear a noise during the concert? Was it annoying?"

Of course most of the students had heard me, but no one answered because they didn't know if they should. They didn't know if it was a joke or not.

Into the silence, Mr. Myer said, "The person making all the noises is Brad Cohen."

I stood up with all kinds of emotions racing through my head. Although I had agreed ahead of time to talk with the entire assembly, now I was realizing that it was going to be harder than I thought. I made the long walk to the front of the room with everyone staring at me because I continued to make noises and tic uncontrollably. When I arrived in front of the hundreds of students, I was nervous, anxious, and very uncomfortable. But I was also very excited. It was like getting a new bicycle and wanting to tell everyone about it—to show people how cool it really was. But this time there was no bicycle. There was just me, and this was my chance to tell everyone why I was making the funny noises and the silly tics all day during class. I really hoped I wouldn't blow it.

When I got to the front, Mr. Myer told the school about Tourette's and that I couldn't help what I did. We stood up there in front of everyone for only about ten minutes, because thirteen- and fourteen-year-olds can absorb only so much information about a disorder they have never heard of before. As my principal explained that I disliked making the noises much more than they disliked hearing them, I felt the crowd relax. And, as I looked out over the many faces in front of me, I realized that I had taken the first small step toward controlling my own destiny.

I had a few more things to say now than I had on the *Sally Jesse Raphael Show*. Also, Mr. Myer and I had discussed this beforehand, so I had had several days to prepare, and this day—the day I had been waiting for for years—couldn't have come soon enough. I was finally going to tell the kids in my school about Tourette's from my viewpoint. Through that, a weight was going to be lifted from my shoulders. I hoped.

Boy, was I nervous. I was sweating bullets that day because it was a day that meant everything to me. The whole school was there, including the students who had talked about me and mocked and pestered me from day one. But I wasn't nervous about what I was going to say. I had practiced, and I was ready.

In the front of the big room, Mr. Myer asked me questions and I answered them as fully as I could. Because Mr. Myer was so well liked, it meant something to all of us when he talked. If he said everyone should listen to what I had to say, well, then, they would listen. He had a very calm, soothing manner, and that made me feel much more comfortable about speaking in front of everyone. Plus, I had spoken at Camp Sabra the summer before, educating the campers and counselors about Tourette's, and that had gone very well.

I had chosen Camp Sabra as the place to make my first speech about my Tourette syndrome because it was a place where I felt completely comfortable. When you are at camp for four weeks, you really get to know people. We ate, slept, played, and lived together all that time. I think camp friends form a special bond that is difficult to explain unless you've experienced it yourself. Essentially, those were the people who knew me better than anyone, except my mom and Jeff.

There, and here at school, I told people that Tourette syndrome is a neurological disorder that causes me to make noises and tics that I can't control. I had memorized those words from a brochure I had on Tourette's, so that part was fairly easy.

"You will notice that I—woop, woop—make my noises more when I am nervous, uncomfortable, under stress, in a new situation—RAH, rah, rah—and when I think about it," I said. "But when I am relaxed, not stressed, or around people I know, I—fa, FA . . . woop—will not do it as much. I don't want to make—woop—these noises, but there is no cure at this—woop, woop—time, so this is what I do."

Mr. Myer then asked me to share how I felt about having Tourette's. I said it was hard and I only wanted to be treated like everyone else. I also mentioned that I was excited to share this information with them so they could understand why I made all the noises, and I encouraged them to come to me if they had any questions. I assured them that I was open and honest about my Tourette's, and I was happy to talk with them any time.

As I handed the microphone back to the principal and began walking to my seat, all the people in the room began clapping. I hesitated, but then I realized the applause was for me. I could hardly believe it. Hundreds of kids were clapping for me just because I had gotten up in front of them and educated them about Tourette's. Talk about positive reinforcement—this was it.

Later, Bill Myer reflected on the event: "It seemed an appropriate time to address this because there were some rather quiet passages in the music and I knew everyone had heard Brad during those times, so it would be easy for me to illustrate what I intended to say about Brad and his condition. Even though Brad's mom kept his teachers and me informed [about Tourette's], there was still a lot of ignorance. Some teachers and even more kids mistakenly thought Brad could control 'it' if he tried."

Mr. Myer added that as soon as I entered junior high, there had been a flurry of discussion among the teachers, nurse, social worker, director of special education, and others on staff trying to find out about Tourette syndrome, what caused it, and how it was addressed. "It became part of our professional development," he said. "I know Brad was terribly hurt at times, more so by the fact that nothing could be done to 'fix' it. When that happened, my philosophy was that there were only a couple of things we could do: educate people and counsel Brad in such a way that he understood and could steel himself against others. I cannot imagine what it was like for him."

✳ ✳ ✳

I realize now that after my Bar Mitzvah, my self-esteem got its next big boost the day I gave my presentation at Camp Sabra. Next came the *Sally Jesse Raphael Show*. My self-esteem rose even more after my speech to my school. I felt like I had been wearing a mask to school every day, and that speech was the equivalent of ripping it off. At last my classmates could see the real me behind the weird kid who barked. Yes, I was a little different, but now the kids all knew why. They had been told before, but never in a way that made sense—to me or to them. I also think the person who presents information has to believe that the information he or she is giving is factual, and that wasn't always the case when teachers talked to my classmates about Tourette syndrome. If the teachers didn't believe that my tics were uncontrollable, how could I expect the students to believe?

This was also one of the best days of my life because I could now articulate to others what was wrong with me, and I would no longer have to rely on others to speak for me. Before my speech at Camp Sabra the previous summer, and before the *Sally Jesse Raphael Show*, I couldn't really explain Tourette's. Those two incidents were my warm-up for this day. I had been fine-tuning my words all this time, and today I was able to explain Tourette's so it made sense. No longer was I a sympathy case in which people looked at me and said, "Poor kid. I feel sorry for him and his family." No longer was I "Brad Cohen who has Tourette's." For the first time, the kids at school could look past the Tourette's and see me, "Brad Cohen, a pretty good guy who also has Tourette's." The difference in perception was huge.

I quickly learned that I felt much better talking about Tourette's than sitting around letting others talk about me. When the kids clapped for me, it sent a message loud and clear. They appreciated my efforts in educating them, and that, in turn, made me a stronger person. I was quickly seeing that education was a very important factor in my world.

For most people, junior high is the time when puberty hits, and the lives of both boys and girls change physically, emotionally, and socially. My biggest change, however, came in that single day, when I took responsibility for all my actions, controllable or not. My life changed the day I was able to take the initiative and educate others. I felt power in that. It was like a door opening to a brand-new world. I had thought of being an educator before, but until now I had never tasted what that was going to be like. Now this desire was such a strong feeling that it surrounded and embraced me. Someday, some way, I knew—Tourette's or no Tourette's—I was going to be a teacher.

My experience on the stage also gave me a hunger to make more speeches. But that would come later. The rest of the school year was, if not good, much better than the first part of the year. Some kids really did treat me better. A few even became my friends. Now that was a novel experience, having friends—my own friends, not friends who were borrowed temporarily from my brother, but my own friends. All mine. At that point, I was very grateful to anyone who wanted to befriend me, because I knew that in being my friend they were taking a risk, too. To some, I was still the weird kid, and friends of mine were subject to the same taunts and mockery that I was getting. But there were a few brave souls who opened themselves to me, and I welcomed them.

The importance of friendship cannot be overestimated. Our friends give us support, confidence, shared experiences, and balance. They are people we play with, laugh with, cry with, and even fight with. Imagine your life without all that, and it is a very bleak existence indeed. So you can see why I felt in a way as if I were in that scene in *The Wizard of Oz* where Dorothy steps from the black-and-white farmhouse into the colorful Land of Oz.

I don't want to give the impression that because of the speech I was suddenly Mr. Popularity. That wasn't the case at all. Not everyone accepted me, and I still had problems with a few teachers. But up to this point in my life, I had embraced Tourette's as my best—and only—friend. Now it was nice to welcome a few others into my world. Tourette's was still there, but the door was open for others to join me; through them, I gained a whole world of new experiences.

The speech had opened the floodgates. I had a lot of catching up to do, physically, emotionally, and socially—and I had only a few more months to do it in. High school was just around the corner.

6

THE INVITATION

PARKWAY CENTRAL HIGH SCHOOL had about sixteen hundred students. The first few days were kind of scary because I was the new kid—along with four hundred other freshmen. But the fear was good because it leveled the playing field with the other freshmen. We had something in common.

What we did not have in common was the locations of our lockers. For some reason, school administrators thought it would be better if I had my locker in a different hall, separated from the other freshmen. Why they thought separating me from my classmates—making me walk to a different hallway and physically distancing myself from them—would be better, I have no clue. But that's the way it was. The location didn't really bother me except that sometimes I had to load up on books for several classes at once, as I couldn't get back to my locker after every class. On the plus side, I had a whole locker to myself, while most kids had to share a locker. They often had to buy special shelving to make room for two sets of books, two coats, and so on. I didn't have that problem.

Now that I was in high school I rode the bus to and from school every day. This was a big switch from previous years. Since the incident in which I got suspended for fighting, I hadn't seen much of the inside of a school bus. So this was a big step—that I could ride on a bus without fear of being beaten up. It showed me how far others had come in accepting me—and my Tourette's.

The morning ride was filled with anticipation of the coming school day, but the afternoon ride often seemed endless. Because it was a constant struggle for me to contain my tics even somewhat during classes, I would be drained from a long day of ticcing and studying. I am never able to totally suppress the tics, and trying makes them a lot worse when I finally *stop* trying. So once I got on the afternoon bus, I would sit alone barking and twitching nonstop. I was also dealing with the general hardships of being a freshman. I ticced more on the bus because I could—it was a more open area than the classroom. Sometimes, when I became uncomfortable or knew I was bothering others, I got off at an earlier stop and faced a long walk home. Better that than to stay on the bus and tic.

Home remained my most comfortable place. Still, many more people across the country had started hearing of Tourette's. The *Sally Jesse Raphael* program had helped tremendously with that. When, in my sophomore year, David E. Kelley devoted an episode of his show *L. A. Law* to a case involving a man with Tourette syndrome, it had an even larger impact on people with TS. Millions of people saw that show—many remember it still—and were able to sympathize with the innocent man who had been stricken with a condition he could not control. The mainstream media's recognition of Tourette syndrome was bringing it forth as a legitimate condition, and that made it infinitely easier for everyone with Tourette's, including me.

Bolstered by increasing media attention to the condition and by my successful speeches at school and at Camp Sabra, I instituted a new policy when I entered high school. I had gained enough confidence that I decided to introduce myself to my new teachers before the semester began. I decided to take the initiative in educating others about TS and not leave anything to chance. Never again did I want to walk into a classroom and have the stress of wondering whether the new teacher would understand Tourette syndrome. Because of my decision, when I entered any of my high school classrooms I knew the teachers understood Tourette's because I had told them all about it. Somewhere along the line I realized that a lot of my teachers didn't know how to talk about Tourette's or how to teach their students about it. By talking with them I was able to help them through this process, and it was easier for everyone concerned.

I also asked each teacher to give me two minutes on the first day of class to explain Tourette's to the other students. Many of the freshmen came from the same junior high that I had attended, so I did know some of the students, and they knew I had TS and what it was. But I also felt a need to educate the upperclassmen. Essentially, I gave the same speech to every class I was in every semester. I didn't care if a student had heard it before. I didn't care if the class had ten students in it or a hundred. I was determined to give that speech. In a way, I thrived on it because the speech got better every time I gave it. And, as time went along, I began to realize that I was indeed making a difference. If someone heard me make the speech a second or even a third time, it rammed the symptoms of Tourette's home that much harder. Some kids even went home and told their parents or mentioned it to kids who weren't in my classes.

My goal in giving the speeches was to help people understand that I had Tourette's, and all that that entailed, but at the same time I wanted them to see that it was not going to stop me from being a student in this particular high school. Also, it was not going to stop me from being their friend.

The other thing my speeches accomplished was, in a very one-sided way, to introduce me to every person in every class. In learning about Tourette's and about me, other students got the feeling that they knew me. This familiarity paved the way to many of my activities in high school and led to some lasting friendships.

There are many differences between junior high school and high school, with one of the biggest being the greater maturity level in high school. In high school, most of the kids were good about learning about Tourette's. So were most of the teachers. For the first time, I felt I could pursue my studies and follow my interests and not have Tourette's get in my way. My freshman year, I worked on the yearbook (and would become coeditor my senior year), joined the racquetball team (in which I eventually earned a varsity letter), took beginning journalism, and continued my Spanish classes. I also began losing weight about this same time, and the early weight loss was encouraged by a new commitment on my part to forego fried foods.

My interest in teaching children also led me to take a child development class as a freshman. It was a good class for me because it was mostly comprised of upperclassmen, so I got to be with many students who had never experienced Tourette's before. One of the more interesting things we had to do for that class was to take care of an egg and pretend that the egg was our baby. I took the job very seriously, even though I was only a freshman. I remember making arrangements with my mom to baby-sit the egg while I was doing other things. I know she thought it was silly, but she supported me in this, as she did in everything I took on. I am proud to report that I took excellent care of my egg!

Following all these different interests was a very positive experience for me because, unlike math class, where I'd go in, take notes, and leave, these classes were interactive. I learned that the more I participated in class, the more the teacher and the students learned not to fear tics and twitches. Little by little, people started jumping on board. They learned that I wasn't so different from them after all, and soon I sensed another reaction that was brand-new to me. It was respect.

✳   ✳   ✳

In November of my freshman year, my life took a definite turn for the better when an older kid named Lenny Minkovich called my house. Lenny was recruiting new members for the B'nai B'rith Youth Organization (BBYO). I was thrilled to receive the invitation because BBYO is a great organization that provides opportunities for Jewish youth to develop leadership potential, and it was something I definitely wanted to explore.

The kids participate in small local groups, known as chapters, under the guidance of adult advisors and professional staff, and work on any number of service projects or activities.

Up until now the JCC—or the "J," as we called it—had been my escape. For years, Jeff and I had been "J-Rats," effectively infiltrating every possible activity we could at the center. For the most part, our experiences at the J were sports oriented, and that was great for active kids such as Jeff and me.

But through the leadership opportunities at BBYO, I found a new second home and the social life I craved. People used to say that BBYO was my life, but that wasn't really true. BBYO actually gave me a life beyond BBYO, in that my life finally changed direction when I started taking on leadership roles. I started as the corresponding secretary for my chapter, a job that involved regularly calling all thirty members and telling them about upcoming activities. It was a tedious job nobody wanted but me because it involved dialing, hoping someone would answer, and explaining the various activity options thirty separate times. This was long before BBYO or any of its local chapters had websites where all that information could be posted online or e-mailed. In that I was lucky, because I knew it was a great opportunity. Just like when I was standing in front of the class at school telling classmates about Tourette's, as I was calling all the BBYO members in my chapter they were learning about me and learning how to interact with my Tourette's.

My friend Al Snyder remembers first meeting me at BBYO when I was continually clearing my throat at meetings. I still stayed in the back of the room whenever I was in a group setting and tried to be as unobtrusive as possible, but people could hear me.

"The throat clearing didn't bother me," Al recalled, "but the laughter that accompanied the noise did. I had no idea that the person making the noise was different from the boys who were laughing. The throat clearing and subsequent laughter made it difficult to concentrate on the meeting, so I looked around the room to find the person making the noise so I could tell him to shut up. I just presumed whoever was making the noise was doing it intentionally. I had not yet met Brad or learned of his disorder, so I was completely unaware that the throat clearing was attributable to Tourette syndrome."

A few weeks later, I helped kill the laughter when I stood up at a BBYO meeting to explain Tourette's. I think Al, along with the others, was astounded.

"I remember being fascinated by Brad's speech," recalled Al. "How could someone have such a disorder? How could I never have heard of it? I had so many questions."

After I finished speaking I opened the floor for questions, and Al was one of the first to raise his hand. He asked if I made the noises when I slept. I laughed and said no, I didn't, because I was so relaxed. That was my first interaction with Al, who was later to become, and remain, a very close friend.

✳ ✳ ✳

Lenny was excited for me to do more in BBYO. He didn't just want me involved. He wanted to see me active. In February, just three months after I joined, he helped me organize a program for the entire St. Louis Council in which I would educate them about Tourette syndrome. This was to be my first official speech in front of a really large group of people. It differed from the two previous times I had spoken to large groups because this was the first time I practiced and prepared actual material that was all my own. I knew exactly what I was going to say, whereas the other times, though I had an idea of what I would say, much of what I said was off-the-cuff, or answers to questions from Mr. Myer or the counselor at Camp Sabra.

Surprisingly, it wasn't difficult. The only reason I was at all nervous at first was because I was a freshman and I was speaking to all ages of high school students. Even the advisors, who were adults, were listening. I was still at the age when being around someone older than me, even by just a few years, both impressed and intimidated me.

I spoke for a time about Tourette syndrome and about my life, and I was amazed to see that everyone was so interested in what I had to say that their eyes stayed on me. I was astounded to realize that I had my audience's attention throughout the entire presentation. People didn't talk to each other and they didn't want to leave. What a contrast with just a year ago, when people's eyes would slide up to me and quickly slide away.

When I was done, people came up to congratulate me. My surprise continued when I learned that they all wanted to talk to me—the entire St. Louis Council for BBYO. Everyone asked questions and I answered them as fast as they were asked. I was excited because not only did everyone now know about Tourette syndrome, they now knew about me.

A few months later, one of the people who had been at the St. Louis Council meeting asked me to speak at a regional

BBYO convention in Omaha, Nebraska. I agreed for two reasons. First, it would give me the opportunity to educate even more people about Tourette's. Second, it would allow me to get to know more people. I was quickly realizing that the more I gave my little speech, the more people knew who I was. If more people knew who I was, then there were more people supporting me. That support was crucial, and something I had been lacking for far too long.

We all need validation from our peers. Imagine spending years sitting in a room full of people who laugh at you every time you blink. You try very hard not to blink, because you know the blinking is annoying others, but before too long you have to blink and so you do blink—several times. Half the people in the room snicker at you, and the other half turn and give you cold stares. As the days and weeks go along, it's hard not to become paranoid and withdrawn. You feel bad about yourself; inside you feel unworthy to be sitting in the same room as these people. Then one day you get up in front of the people who have snickered and stared at you your entire life and explain why you are blinking, and some of the people understand. Not all, but some. You figure if you get up in front of more people then maybe a few more will understand, and they do. Soon, you take every opportunity you can to educate people because you find that the support of the few who understand gives you courage and strength.

In Omaha, I stepped up to the microphone in front of a crowd of well over one hundred people and explained Tourette syndrome. Everyone seemed interested in what I said. After I spoke, I took questions. After I was done, people congratulated me, and I experienced a beautiful rush of success—something I had not felt very many times. It was a wonderful feeling.

From that point on, BBYO was my home, and I knew I was one step closer to my dream of someday being entrusted with a classroom full of children—even though I had no idea how or where that might happen.

✻ ✻ ✻

My success in BBYO was helping me in all areas: friendships, schoolwork, self-esteem, and, most importantly, with my family. My dad and his parents still didn't feel comfortable taking me out to a restaurant, but things were definitely less strained at family gatherings. I think they saw some of the success I was having at BBYO and thought there might be hope for me after all. While some of them still didn't understand Tourette's, they were realizing that maybe I wasn't the lost cause they had thought I was.

One of the things that made family gatherings both better and worse was the presence of my dad's new wife, my stepmother, Diane. Diane had begun to be a part of our lives prior to my Bar Mitzvah, when she and Dad were still dating. In her favor, Diane tried. She did everything right. But as far as Jeff and I were concerned, she wasn't a welcome addition to the family. It wasn't Diane; it was the position she held as Dad's new wife that bothered us. Dad could have married anyone, but no matter who it was we would have resented her.

At the time, we had trouble with the fact that Dad loved someone in addition to us. As difficult and strained as our relationship had been, he was still our dad and we didn't want anyone infringing on his feelings for us. Then there was our loyalty to our mother. We felt we should support her, and one way Jeff and I thought we could do that was to dislike Diane.

On the plus side, Diane served as a sort of intermediary between Dad and myself. She was able to see the family dynamics up close from an outsider's perspective, and that gave her a unique point of view. Looking back, I think Diane was influential in helping Dad deal with my Tourette's. I may not have been the ideal firstborn son he visualized, but some good qualities were emerging and Diane helped my dad see those.

Diane remembers one time just before I entered high school when I visited Dad and Diane in Atlanta. She and I were running an errand, and I for once felt comfortable enough with her to begin talking about my lack of friends.

"I was flattered that Brad confided and opened up to me," recalled Diane. "At the same time, I hoped I was going to say something that would really help and inspire Brad and that I wouldn't blow it. Soon after that Brad became active in BBYO and the involvement made an incredible difference for him. His personality blossomed and he became a very popular leader, and with that came many friends. Over a relatively short time, Brad went from introvert to major-league extrovert. BBYO did so much to broaden his background and build confidence."

A letter from a friend I met in BBYO, Pam Howard, supports the validation I experienced with my involvement in that group.

I always refer to Brad as "my hero." I really admired his self-confidence, his courage, and his determination to do everything he wanted to do despite his tics and the terrible way he was treated. I was so impressed that he stood in front of hundreds of people and spoke about his tics in a way that made people feel comfortable around him. He always had a sense of humor about it and was always willing to answer other people's questions. Brad always made me feel very good about myself and very comfortable being me, and I never felt judged or criticized by him; instead I was, and still am, inspired.

BBYO helped me in so many ways, especially with my confidence. BBYO came along at exactly the right time in my life. That was good because in the coming years, as I faced the challenges of entering adulthood with Tourette's, I was going to need every bit of confidence I could muster.

7

WHEN THE "THING" WINS

I BASKED IN A NORMAL HIGH SCHOOL LIFE, one that included friends, the yearbook staff, and the racquetball team. Finally, I had reached a level of acceptance at school that included a table in the cafeteria where I could sit and talk and laugh with friends while we all ate lunch. Just one year earlier, that simple thing was a fantasy. Of additional help was the fact that in my sophomore year, my principal from junior high school, Mr. Myer, moved up to the high school. It was wonderful to have support at his level. But while the students and teachers who were regularly in my school understood my Tourette's and me, those who were not regulars often treated me unfairly.

One day we had a substitute teacher in one of my high school classes, and it was a day that my tics were especially bad. I assumed that the sub had been told about my tics, but apparently that was not the case. It didn't help that this particular substitute had no patience with kids. She kept asking me to be quiet, even though I told her I had Tourette's and couldn't control my outbursts. There was still nothing worse than sitting in class and having a teacher ridicule me over what I couldn't control. I felt embarrassed and helpless.

I apologized several times for interrupting the class, but she sent me to the principal's office anyway. Because I was banished in the middle of things and didn't witness the rest of the events, I'll let my friend Eric Ludwig finish the story.

"I remember this incident very well," Eric recalled, "because it was really an eye-opener for me to see the way some people treated Brad, and this substitute was particularly rude and insensitive. I knew Brad had to deal with some crazy things, but I never thought it would come from a member of the faculty. After Brad left, some of the other class members and I really gave it to the sub, really brought her to tears. We were livid. I felt bad about going off on the sub, but then I thought of how Brad must have felt and how he has to deal with this kind of treatment regularly."

The fiasco with the substitute teacher was just one illustration of why I still did not like to go out in public—I didn't know how strangers would react. Not that I was housebound or anything, but I did not go often to places you might go regularly—places such as the grocery store, the mall, the movie theater, or the library. TS didn't totally stop me from going to public places, but the difficult part of being in public was the unpredictability—not knowing what might happen or how people might treat me. Tourette syndrome continued to get in my way. It got me kicked out of restaurants and movies. During these times my friends, like Eric, stuck up for me, which made me feel really good. After years of no peer support, I was especially grateful for it now.

One Friday night some friends and I went to a local restaurant called Tippins for some pie. As we tried to order, the manager told me I had to stop making noises or I would be asked to leave, so I gave him my standard spiel about Tourette's: "Hi. I'm Brad, and the noises and tics I am making are because I have Tourette syndrome. Tourette syndrome is a neurological disorder that causes me to make noises and tics I can't control. I'm really open and honest about Tourette syndrome, so if you have any questions, please feel free to ask. Thank you."

After hearing my explanation, he seemed to understand and he left. But not for long. A few minutes later he very loudly told us we would need to move into a corner because I was disturbing people. It was a very awkward moment. It wasn't so much what the manager asked us to do; it was the way he asked. He was very defensive and loud and turned the situation into a public scene.

Usually when I go out in public and someone asks about Tourette's, I'll gladly educate him or her. Then, if the person still doesn't understand, my friends jump in. I've never talked with my friends about jumping in—it's just something they do spontaneously, and usually with far more passion than I. You see, I am used to these situations. They are not. So when something like this happens, my friends get frustrated and defend me.

You might wonder how I feel during all this. Well, I am embarrassed for myself and for whomever I am with. I revert back to the kid I was in junior high, and I become afraid that my friends won't want to do things with me anymore. I know I am not doing anything wrong, yet I am being punished. It is a terrible and depressing feeling, to say the least. Invariably, the person kicking me out of wherever we are becomes increasingly arrogant. My chance of educating the individual about Tourette's, and thus finding a positive outcome to the problem, decreases as his or her level of arrogance increases. I fully understand that my noises can be distracting to others, and I am willing to compensate by doing whatever I can to help out. All I ask is that I be treated with the same courtesy and respect that the person who is distracted is receiving.

In this case, in addition to being kicked out, we were publicly humiliated. We tried to enjoy the rest of the evening, but the damage had been done; our evening had been spoiled. Now all we could talk about was "the situation." I didn't mind, but I figured we could have been talking about other, more enjoyable things if only the manager had been more pleasant. But it didn't happen that way. I was very upset, mostly because the whole scene need not have happened.

Talk about timing—the next morning our newspaper printed an article about another guy in the area who had Tourette's. I decided to take action. I called Tippins headquarters in Kansas City and I sent them the article. The company executives were so apologetic that they ended up sending me a gift certificate for my friends and me to have a complimentary meal. I was pleased that they did the right thing. One of their employees messed up, but they did what they could to make amends. The best thing of all? There was no dollar amount on the certificate. We could order as much as we wanted.

The first chance we got, I rounded up my friends and we ordered a feast. I, personally, made sure I had two pieces of pie. Sometimes there are advantages to having Tourette's.

"We ran up a huge bill that night," recalled David Amsterdam, one of my friends who was with me on both occasions. "But on the first night we had gotten a bunch of dirty looks from the manager and the other customers, and we were treated badly. We all felt they owed us, and the second time we made sure we had a lot of fun."

✳   ✳   ✳

The other good news was that all around me I was raising consciousness of TS, and things continued to improve with my family. No, we hadn't turned into the family on *Leave It to Beaver* or anything, but I could see definite progress. Once in a while, as a family, we could even share a laugh.

One night I was having dinner at my aunt Laurie and uncle Stu's. I was really ticcing that day, going hard and heavy every few seconds with "Ja, JA . . . JA" and "Woop, woop." My cousin Mandy was six or seven then, and as soon as I made a noise she would imitate me. Then their dog, Pepper, would bark. So there we all were at the dinner table.

"Woop, woop."

"Woop, woop."

"Aarf."

"Woop, woop."

"Woop, woop."

"Aarf."

Laurie later recalled, "Stu and I were mortified that Mandy was imitating Brad. But then we all looked at each other and burst out laughing—Brad included—because it was so funny with Pepper barking."

The incident became a learning session for Mandy as Laurie and Stu later explained to her that I couldn't keep from making the noises, and she got her first real lesson on Tourette's. A few years later when Mandy was making her Bat Mitzvah, she gave a donation to the Tourette Syndrome Association as her charitable gift. I was incredibly touched by her gesture because much more than the monetary gift, it validated Tourette's, and me, in that part of our family.

Those were the good times. But sometimes everything was so grim that all I could do was cry. One of the lowest moments in my life came when I got my first job as a busboy at a popular restaurant. By this time I had turned sixteen and had recently gotten my driver's license, a momentous occasion in the life of most teens, but especially in mine. My parents never put pressure on me to get a job, but it was something I really wanted. Ever since I was little, I had loved taking on responsibilities and helping out others. I would mow lawns, shovel snow, or baby-sit. I didn't do it for money; I just liked helping out. But now that I had a driver's license I thought about doing something that would actually pay.

One afternoon my friend Al and I applied at Marciano's Restaurant. The manager interviewed us, and to our great delight we were immediately hired as busboys. We each quickly found some black pants and a white shirt—our uniform—and we reported later that day for work.

I can't tell you how happy I was to have this job. I was going to be clearing tables. I was so excited. It sounds strange to be so thrilled about such a menial job, but being in the workforce was something I had been looking forward to for a long time.

Then, standing there in uniform, even before I started my job, I was fired. Even though I had told the manager when he was interviewing me that I had Tourette syndrome and he hired me anyway, I was fired. He said that on further thought he had decided that I would disturb the customers.

I was devastated, and Al was as upset as I was. He offered to quit, but I encouraged him to stay. There was no point in both of us being jobless. I went out to my car and got in, and the tears began to flow. I was so disappointed and hurt and angry. I wondered if Tourette's would keep me from ever having a job—if I would ever be able to support myself. I wondered if my dream of being the teacher that I never had was just a delusion. I wondered why I had to go through all this, why I had to endure being mocked and beaten up and rejected time after time, day after day. It was one of the few times I have given in and let Tourette's take over. It was one of the few times I have just plain given up. I cried so hard all the way home it's a wonder I got there safely.

When I got home I shut myself in my bedroom and cried so hard my mother had to kick the door down to get to me. Now I have to smile at the image of my tall, thin mom breaking down the door. It was the ultimate display of a parent protecting her child. But at the time I couldn't find any humor in the situation. At that moment, I really needed my mom. I was truly a broken man.

*   *   *

My parents and I sued the restaurant for firing me. This was in the early 1990s, right around the time Congress passed the Americans with Disabilities Act (ADA), a federal civil rights law that prohibits discrimination against people with disabilities in everyday activities, including work-related situations. I found a copy of the law, cut it out, and put it in my wallet. It also said that a public place must make reasonable accommodations for a disabled person. I liked these words, and this law in my pocket would become good ammunition in the future. I would just pull it out and show people that they couldn't kick me out of a restaurant or a movie. They had to provide me a reasonable accommodation. This tactic has usually worked.

We hired a lawyer, who argued that the restaurant had violated the ADA. The courts ended up being favorable to me and I won a small settlement. That was gratifying, but what I really wanted was a part-time job like a regular teenager. At this time and in this place, however, it was not to be. The experience reinforced a hard but valuable lesson—that there were going to be limitations in my life, limitations made by others that I could not control.

That's the way it goes when the "thing" wins. Sometimes you can't take the straight path; you have to find your own way. But my life with Tourette's has made me realize that everyone has a "thing" that haunts them in some way. It might be prejudice or chronic illness. It might be physical limitations or life circumstances or ego or pride or jealousy or hate, but everyone has their thing. When we can control the thing, we feel empowered and optimistic. But when the thing wins, we travel the road to despair. The key is to find a road that leads around your particular limitation, a road that maybe has more bends in it but gets you to the same point in the end.

Once I realized that, I understood all the more that my road in the workplace was going to be traveled with young kids. Before they are taught differently, kids do not judge. They do not criticize unless they are encouraged to do so by their families and peers. Generally, children are open and curious and loving, and I wanted to be the teacher who encourages those traits. Somehow I knew I'd get there.

* * *

Within a few years, I had taken on more responsibility in BBYO and eventually was twice elected president of the St. Louis Council. In that capacity—and other BBYO positions—I traveled across the United States. Each time I got elected to a new office, my name and sometimes my photo would run in the local paper. I eventually had the honor of being one of ten people elected from around the world to the BBYO International Board, a position that held a great deal of accountability and required some international travel. This was huge!

The election to an international position took place in Pennsylvania during my senior year in high school. After the election I flew home and was greeted at the airport by my mom and Jeff . . . and by my dad! I thought it was a bit odd that Dad was in town, because we still did not see him that often, but as soon as we got to my house, I found out why. All my friends had gathered to celebrate my big victory. In that moment, I realized I wasn't alone in winning the international position; all my friends, my family, and the St. Louis Council had won, too. They were my team—my support group—and they all played a big part in helping me achieve everything that I had achieved.

Everyone was so excited for me, and I was excited for them. They all wanted to hear the details about the election and my trip and my new responsibilities. Everyone wanted to share the excitement.

"You really had to be there to understand how happy we were for Brad," said Jeff. "We were in the middle of witnessing this amazing transformation my brother was going through. One reason we were so excited is that we all kept thinking of Brad just a few years before—the overweight, out-of-control kid with no social skills. Now he was on the international board of BBYO. Amazing."

Steve Mathes agreed. "So many people give BBYO the credit for Brad's success," he said, "but I really think it was Brad himself. BBYO helped, certainly, but Brad has an incredible amount of drive and determination. Without his never-say-no attitude, with or without Tourette syndrome, none of this would have happened."

In my new position I planned conventions, participated in conference calls, traveled the world, and met some very neat people across the globe. I can't say what the best part of all of it was, but traveling and meeting people from around the world has to be one of the highlights. I met so many people who are still friends of mine to this day. It was just an incredible experience, and pretty good for a kid who a few short years earlier couldn't even find someone to sit with in the lunchroom. (If I'm repeating myself, it's a sign of how much my new life really meant to me.)

My first international trip was to Poland. Traveling, for obvious reasons, can be difficult. Often, people stare. In fact, the number of people who turn to look at me in an airport is amazing. It's a very weird feeling. I feel their eyes on me, and it makes it hard for me to concentrate on anything else, so one of my strategies is to just stare back. It doesn't exactly lighten up the situation for anybody, but it makes me feel better and hopefully it makes some people realize what they are doing. I know my Tourette's often makes me the center of attention, but some people seem to think that I'm their own personal freak show.

I can't avoid flying on airplanes. Like everyone else, I have places to go, and when I fly I always get a mixed bag of reactions—compassion and disgust, confusion and irritation. I sometimes wish I could get up in front of the passengers and make my speech like I did in my classroom at school.

I always try to prepare myself mentally before I get to the plane, and when I step on board I sometimes tell the flight attendants that I have Tourette's. But sometimes I don't. It all depends on the situation and how I feel at the time. If I tell the flight staff, I usually pull away from my brother or whomever I am traveling with so they aren't bothered with my problem. I never want to put the burden of my Tourette's on people I am flying with. If I am really calm and relaxed, then I might not say anything to the flight staff at all.

If I have a long flight, I do my best to relax. Because I don't tic when I am asleep, it's an easier ride for everyone if I sleep part or all of the way.

Most of the time I tell people who are sitting close to me about Tourette's. Many times they nod and accept it without a problem. But it's not uncommon for some people to ask the flight attendant if they can move to a new seat. Although they never say it directly, I can tell by their body language that they want to move to get away from me. That used to bother me—a lot—but now I realize that they are just uneducated about Tourette's and feel uncomfortable, so it's okay.

I've actually learned to enjoy watching how different people talk about me. It's a real study in human nature. Most try to be polite and talk in a way that they think I won't notice. But I live with Tourette's day in and day out. I have excellent peripheral vision and I can read lips. I can sense what is going on and I can tell when people are talking about me by the way they start whispering and the way they casually lean over and look at me. Again, it's okay, especially if I've told one of them I have Tourette's. I understand that they are just educating each other, and it makes me feel better if I know someone understands rather than having them look over at me a million times and asking themselves, "What in the world is he doing?" If they are just staring and pointing and being openly rude, I might even go up to them and talk to them about Tourette's.

In Poland, there were over a hundred of us BBYO teens. We were all representing our respective cities as part of a BBYO Holocaust education program known as the March of the Living. There, upon our after-midnight arrival, I had my first opportunity to speak about Tourette's on foreign soil.

"Our group was gathered at the Forum Hotel in Warsaw," recalled Jeremy Poock, a friend I met on the trip. "We were all so tired, as we had traveled from New York, and our advisors were giving us instructions for the next day. Through it all, I kept hearing these strange noises, although I couldn't tell who or where the noises were coming from. Then Brad was introduced.

Standing in front of complete strangers, Brad explained that he had Tourette syndrome and that the noises we heard were caused by his condition. My reaction was pure admiration. I admired Brad for his courage to speak up in front of us all. And I admired him because I knew even then that Brad would never let Tourette's get in the way of pursuing any endeavor he wished to pursue."

From the moment I gave my speech, I had no trouble on that trip, or any other that BBYO sponsored. I also noticed that although there was somewhat of a language barrier wherever I traveled, once I explained what Tourette's was all about, most people in other countries were more accepting of it than people here in the United States. I know I gained more friends and life experience during my stint in BBYO than in any other endeavor I have been a part of.

✳ ✳ ✳

During my junior year of high school, most of my peers were deciding where to go to college. Schoolwork was so hard for me that I didn't like thinking about college and all the reading I would have to do. But I knew that if I were going to be a teacher, to college I would have to go. One day a voice came over the school intercom announcing that recruiters were visiting that day from Yale, the University of Missouri, and other colleges. One was from Bradley University in Peoria, Illinois. My given name is Bradley and so I thought this might be a perfect match. I met with the recruiter and when she told me that Bradley had a great education major, I decided that was where I would go.

I went home and told my mom and then my dad that I would be going to Bradley University. They both had the same reaction: "You can't go to a school just because it has the same name as you do!" But after I showed them the literature and explained that it was the perfect school for me because of the location (not too far from St. Louis) and the great hands-on education major, they slowly came around. Although they had trouble with my choice at first, it was probably the easiest post-secondary college decision made by any student in history.

But by my senior year, I didn't know if I would be going straight to college from high school. I had risen so high in the B'nai B'rith Youth Organization that I decided to run for president of BBYO, a job that would require me to delay college for a year, travel, and make speeches. I was particularly excited about the possibility of this job because it would put me in a wonderful position to help the organization that had so greatly helped me.

I campaigned hard throughout the summer, and that was a fantastic experience in itself. I had a lot of supporters, but in the end I didn't win the election. Was I upset? Absolutely. I ran to win. But I came in second and had a very positive experience in running my campaign. Looking back, I know things happen for a reason and now I am glad that I lost the election. My entire life could have gone in a different direction if I had won. I had given BBYO everything I could, and the organization had been extremely helpful to me in so many ways. BBYO had given me all the tools I needed to be successful in life. But now, I knew it was time to move on.

Disappointed, but excited to start college, I left for Bradley University, a school that literally had my name all over it. Bradley Cohen attending Bradley University had become a reality.

8

TESTING THE WATERS:
STUDENT TEACHING

BECAUSE OF THE BBYO ELECTION, my transition into college happened very quickly. Until the election was over, I didn't know whether I was going to take the year off from school or report to Bradley University. So after the election, I had to switch gears quickly. I was home in St. Louis for just one day before I was off to Peoria, Illinois.

I was both nervous and excited about this big change. I felt good about being at Bradley, but there was so much to do to get ready. One of those things was to introduce myself to my roommate—a guy named Dave VanDixhorn. A month or so earlier, I had received a letter from Bradley University giving me Dave's name and address. He was from Sheboygan, Wisconsin, and he was a few years older than I was.

In addition to discussing things like who was going to bring the TV and who was going to bring the fridge, I needed to tell Dave about my Tourette's, so in the middle of my BBYO campaign I had called him. I began by asking if he knew what

Tourette syndrome was. He said no and I filled him in. It was a scary call for me because it was something that could have gone very poorly. Fortunately, Dave said he was fine with it. I certainly hoped so, because even though he said everything was fine, there was something in his voice that made me think Dave didn't really understand what an adventure rooming with me was going to be. But when I arrived at Bradley, Dave and I hit it off right away. It was lucky for Dave that I don't tic in my sleep.

Our dorm room was on the sixth of ten floors in Geisert Hall. This was not a building where a lot of freshmen lived, but I chose it for its air-conditioning and for the computer that came with each room. This was a few years before students needed to arrive on campus with their own computer. Dave and I had a lot in common, including that both of us were education majors. We also had differences, including that he had spent the past few years playing baseball at a small California school, and he was a team mascot for Bradley—something I had always thought would be a lot of fun. Dave was easygoing and had a great personality. Our room was small but we had a window with a view of a shopping mall, and we had all the necessities, including a microwave. I slept on the top bunk and life was good.

Going to college pretty much scared me to death; there were so many people from so many places! I had planned to take my high school approach of talking with my teachers ahead of time about Tourette's and then standing in front of the class the first day and explaining Tourette's to the other students. But something happened that changed my plans. Just days after I arrived at Bradley, I unintentionally became a celebrity.

The first week we were all there, everyone was getting to know each other. Classes had not yet started, but fraternity rush was taking place and I was participating in that. A few guys who lived on my floor asked me if I was interested in getting some lunch across the street at the Steak & Fries. I had seen one of the guys around, but I didn't really know him or his friends.

As we were placing our orders, I was making piercing noises like "Fa, fa . . . FA, fa . . . DRA!" along with an occasional "Woop . . . woop!" and my neck was jerking a bit as well. The Steak & Fries employee behind the counter thought I was drunk and told me I had to stop making noises or he would not take my order. Then he threatened to call the police. My new friends stuck up for me as I was trying to explain Tourette's to the man. But he didn't listen and he wouldn't serve us. I was mortified. Here I was at a new school with new friends and we had just gotten kicked out of a restaurant. I hadn't even been there a week. The others said not to worry about it—we could just go to Subway—but I was so disgusted I went back to my room instead.

As soon as I got there I couldn't help but cry. I felt so alone and upset and frustrated. I couldn't believe what had just happened. Classes hadn't even started and I had already been brought to my knees. I wondered—once again—if Tourette's would always keep me from leading a normal life. Would I forever be ejected from places other people enjoyed every day? Would I constantly be judged on my tics and twitches, rather than on who I was behind all that? I was totally distraught—this was definitely not the way I had envisioned starting my new life.

But after my tears dried, my frustration turned to anger. I tried to deal with the situation on my own, but eventually I broke down and called my mom and then my dad. Mom offered to come get me if that's what I wanted, but I wanted to stay. I knew I had to tough it out by myself. It was just a low moment and I needed some support in getting through it.

Then the magic happened—people from my floor began coming to my room. They had heard what had happened. I downplayed it as much as I could, but soon people from other dorms were calling and stopping by. E-mail was fairly new at the time but everyone had an e-mail address. Within hours, e-mails were flying across campus and everyone was talking about me being thrown out of Steak & Fries. Some students—against my wishes—started a boycott of the restaurant. Others even told Steak & Fries management that they were getting the entire student population to boycott the place because of the discrimination the clerk had shown against me.

It didn't take too many kids threatening a boycott before the manager of the Steak & Fries called me. As I looked out my dorm room window at the shopping mall across the street, I could actually see the guy who was on the phone with me. Of course, he didn't know I was watching him, and considering the circumstances I didn't feel the need to fill him in. He was pacing up and down and his hands were flapping—a sure sign of extreme agitation. I could tell just by his voice, though, that he was nervous and he knew they had messed up. He invited me over to the restaurant so he could apologize in person, but I didn't want to go back there. The place was ruined for me. But he kept asking and I finally gave in.

When I arrived, he said he was extremely sorry about what had happened and gave some sad excuse for the person who had thrown me out. He also gave me a handful of coupons for free sandwiches. I accepted them, and his apology, with as much graciousness and dignity as I could muster.

I was so very tired of getting kicked out of public places. It was humiliating and I didn't deserve any of it. This was not the first time my "woop" and "rah, rah" barking noises, my strange facial grimaces, my neck jerks, and all the rest had led people to believe I was drunk or stoned, and probably it wouldn't be the last. But how I wished that this particular incident had never happened. At the same time, I was amazed and excited about the show of support from my new school. It was far more than I had ever imagined and was truly the silver lining in all this. Because everyone on campus had heard about the incident, everyone felt that they knew me. I had instant friends and it was wonderful. So in that sense, I was almost glad it had happened.

The next week *The Bradley Scout*, our university newspaper, ran a story about the incident. It was the first of several articles the newspaper staff would run, and they had a field day with it. Front-page stories accompanied by editorials took the franchise owner to task for allowing an employee to discriminate against someone with a disability. I hope it made the people at Steak & Fries understand that even though someone might be a little different, they still had to treat that person with respect.

I gave some of the coupons to the people who were with me when I was ejected, shared some with a few new friends I had made, and used the rest myself. The day I ran out of coupons was the last day I set foot in a Steak & Fries restaurant.

I didn't care what the other students did. I just made a personal decision not to go back. And I never have.

✳ ✳ ✳

Despite the problem with Steak & Fries, my fellow students' show of support encouraged me, and I continued my participation in rush week. The way it worked at Bradley was that you had to go to all twenty fraternities, then wait and see who wanted you. Hopefully some of the ones you wanted to join were also some of the ones who wanted you. There were three rounds of this, so it was kind of nerve-wracking. I was fortunate and was able to join Alpha Epsilon Pi (AEPi), a national Jewish fraternity. I thought this would be a good option for me, especially because I had been so active in BBYO. AEPi did turn out to be an excellent choice, as it gave me a big group of friends to bond with and a great social life. I was selected as pledge-class president (freshman president) of AEPi, and would later become president of my entire Bradley fraternity.

My fraternity activities got me back to what I was good at doing—organizing events and getting people fired up. Everyone in my fraternity accepted Tourette's right away; it was never an issue for anyone. I don't know if the stories in the newspaper helped with that, but whatever the reason, this acceptance took a lot of pressure off me. My fraternity connections also proved to be a good way to meet people, and I soon became well connected throughout the Bradley campus.

Classes did eventually start, and with the exception of one professor who asked me not to sit in the front of the class as my noises distracted him, everything was going great. I sat down with Celia Johnson, my advisor, right away and planned out my next four years as an education major.

My very first semester I was quite pleased to be in a classroom working with fourth-graders at a school close to Bradley. I was only there two hours a day, three days a week, but the point was to get my feet wet and see some real teaching being done. I really enjoyed it and took lots of notes. I was fortunate to be working with a wonderful teacher, because she was modeling what I planned to be doing in just four short years. In fact, all the teachers whose classes I worked in as a student—including Helen Ferguson my junior year and Christina Brock-Lammers my senior year—were superb mentors, and I still keep in touch with many of them.

I loved working with the kids. Being in the classroom was so much better than I had ever dreamed it could be. I really couldn't believe I was finally here! I have always been a hands-on kind of guy. I've never liked practicing or learning the theory behind something; I've always liked doing. So actually getting to be in the classroom working with kids was the beginning of the realization of my lifelong dream.

As the semesters passed, I assisted in a number of classrooms. By my junior year I was in a second grade class three days a week for half a day; and for one semester of my senior year, I was full time in a class of fifth-graders. The school settings ranged from middle-class suburbs to the depths of the inner city, and the children ranged from gifted students to students with resource needs. I really liked that Bradley's education program gave me a wide variety of hands-on experiences. I felt I was being well prepared for just about any possible teaching situation.

Every time I went into a new classroom, I would first talk to the teacher about Tourette's. I was pleased to find that every teacher was pleasantly understanding and committed to me as a future teacher. It was solid validation and very welcome. Then the first day I was in class I'd educate the kids with a question-and-answer session. I explained that Tourette syndrome was a disorder that made me make strange faces and noises that I couldn't help. As usual, I likened it to sneezing or blinking—you know it's coming and you can stall it a little bit, but eventually you're going to sneeze (or blink).

I also explained my Banana Theory to the kids: you can't judge a banana by the outside. The outside of the banana might be all bruised and discolored and look really nasty, but once you open the banana and peel the skin back, there could be a nice, clean, fresh banana inside. I also explained that there are all different kinds of bananas, just as there are all different kinds of people, and that we shouldn't judge either the people or the bananas in our lives until we have the chance to "peel back the skin" and learn what's inside.

Becky Erdman, who was a student teacher at the same time I was, told me she was amazed at how easily the kids understood and accepted my explanations. I've always found that kids generally have no trouble understanding the Banana Theory, and it helps them understand and accept Tourette's. It's too bad the concept is not as easy for adults to grasp.

While I absolutely loved student teaching, there were some things I had not anticipated. I didn't realize how tired I would get. Teachers are on their feet constantly. The level of preparation for the lessons is unbelievable. It is extremely difficult to challenge the students who are doing well and to help the ones who are having trouble, all at the same time, in the same lesson plan. I had not imagined the great amount of time I would have to spend on classroom management and on discipline. Even in my student teaching days, I was never quick to give a time-out or to remove a child from the class. I remembered very well what it was like to be the kid in the corner. I knew how awful that felt, so I tried very hard to understand the reasons for a child's behavior. I believe that if I can find the true underlying cause of the behavior, I can find a way to modify it. Kids need to know that adults care. Once they realize that you care, they are more likely to behave well, or to tell you why they are having trouble.

While I was often busy in the classroom, I still maintained a high level of activity outside my studies. In addition to the responsibilities I had taken on with my fraternity, I also joined Hillel, an organization for Jewish students. Hillel offered a place where you could practice religious activities or take part in the organization's many social events. It was a great place to meet people, and by now you should have figured that out about me: I love to meet people. I did my typical overachiever thing there, too, and ended up president.

One aspect of Hillel that I especially enjoyed was organizing community awareness events. One event I organized was a Holocaust Remembrance Week. During the week, we held a multiday round-the-clock reading of the names of many of the six million Jews who died in that horrific time. Remembering them that way was extremely moving, as the names became very personal to us.

I was particularly invested in organizing the Remembrance Week because of my BBYO trip to Poland. My traveling companions and I had visited the sites of former concentration camps and then traveled on to Israel, where we met and talked with camp survivors. The trip was an eye-opening experience for me, and seeing the camps and talking one-on-one with the survivors made me want to do my part to ensure that nothing like that ever happened again. After we returned to our homes, all of us who had gone on the trip spent time educating our local communities. I wanted to continue educating people about the Holocaust, and the Remembrance Week activities were one way I could accomplish that.

✳ ✳ ✳

My sophomore and junior years I lived in the frat house, and I loved living there. No one seemed to mind a guy who jerked and twitched and barked all day long. I had some concern that once they saw a little more of me, as they would after I moved in, Tourette syndrome would become a problem. But it never did. Not once. Through AEPi, I also became involved in the Interfraternal Council, which oversaw all the fraternities at Bradley. My junior year, I was honored to be elected vice president of this council. Despite my early fears that I wouldn't be able to handle college work because of all the head and neck jerking associated with Tourette's, I was thriving on collegiate life. My grades were great, my social life was wonderful, and I couldn't have been any happier.

During my junior year, the Peoria newspaper did a two-page story on me. It focused on my Tourette's, and my being both a student at Bradley and a future teacher. The story got the attention of many people in the central Illinois area, and the response was unbelievable. There were so many people who knew someone with Tourette's. What a difference from the time I did the *Sally Jesse Raphael Show*, when Tourette syndrome was still virtually unheard of. A lot of education had been done in the past eight years, and I hoped I had had a part in that.

As people who knew of someone with Tourette's or who had Tourette's themselves read the article and called for advice, I kept track of the names and numbers. So many people needed help, especially children in school. To this day, whenever anyone contacts me to learn more about Tourette syndrome, I always take the time. It is my way of giving back. I can't always help the people who have helped me, but I can help others. If I can help make the life of a child easier, maybe prevent him or her from experiencing some of the things I did, then I have done well. I can't tell you how important this has become to me.

Because of the tremendous response from the article, I decided to start a Tourette syndrome support group in Peoria. I remembered my first experience with a support group—the small dark room where everyone was very negative and depressed, and where few were trying to lead normal public lives. That meeting had turned into a series of pessimistic complaints. I vowed that for everyone involved this time, the experience would be different. I wanted to show people that while there were limitations involved in having Tourette's, they could still have a full, fun, and productive life.

At our first meeting we had ten people in the group. At the next meeting there were fifteen, and then there were twenty. It was really interesting for me because many of the people came from rural areas and had never met anyone else with Tourette's before. At first they all just stared at me, but soon the questions started and I was drilled from all sides—by kids and parents alike.

After a few meetings I planned a social for the members with their families. About fifty of us went bowling, and everyone had a really good time. It was also a fundraiser for the group and we did extremely well. Today, I am very proud to say that this support group is still going strong in central Illinois.

* * *

The summer between my junior and senior years at Bradley, I needed to find something to do. The previous summer I had taken a trip to Europe with other Bradley students for class credit. It was a culturally rich program that included visiting castles, museums, casinos, clubs, and other attractions, and I wanted to do something equally as fun—if not quite as exciting—this summer. I had a friend who was going to Emory University and another who had an internship at CNN. Both friends—Jordan Hirschfield and Bob Steinback—were located in Atlanta, as was my dad. I had no idea what I would do in Atlanta, but one of my friends suggested that I could be a counselor at a kids' day camp. A few days later, after just a few phone calls, I was hired over the phone as a counselor at Camp Alterman. So I loaded up the old Volvo that my dad had handed down to me, and headed southeast.

I was excited about being a counselor, but I had a bit of a nagging fear that it wouldn't work out because of my tics. When

I got there, it turned out that the staff members were already familiar with Tourette syndrome because they had another counselor with Tourette's. That was a big relief. Other than my usual two-minute speech on Tourette's, I didn't have to explain myself to anyone, and I threw myself headlong into the summer.

Each week at Camp Alterman the staff members chose a Counselor of the Week, and the very first week I was surprised to be selected. All the unit heads, plus the camp director, voted on who would be chosen, so it was a real peer-voted honor. At the end of the year I was even more pleased to be chosen as Camp Alterman's Counselor of the Year. I kind of felt like the new guy who came in and stole the show, but I can't tell you how much I appreciated the award. Awards to me are like the icing on the cake for doing a great job—never necessary, but always nice.

On another level, awards are important to me. For people to see past the Tourette's and see me, they often need a reason. An award gives them one, and often puts me back on a par with everyone else out there. Plus, it's one thing when one person chooses a winner; it says a lot more when, as with this award, your peers choose you.

That summer, the three of us—Jordan, Bob, and I—shared a small apartment. During the day I was a camp counselor, but in the evenings I got to know the city of Atlanta, and I fell in love with it. My friends and I went out almost every night, and we thoroughly enjoyed all that the city had to offer. I began to think I might want to relocate to Atlanta after I graduated, so in my few free moments I even scoped out some schools that might hire me as a teacher.

Another plus for Atlanta was that Georgia had reciprocity with Illinois for teaching certificates, while Missouri did not. If I moved back to St. Louis, I would have to take another twelve hours of classes before I could be certified there. I was, excited just to be even thinking about these things. I was exhilarated to think that in a little more than a year, I might finally have my own classroom.

* * *

Much of my senior year at Bradley was spent searching for a job, but I was also busy with a new responsibility. Since my freshman year, I had been attending the annual AEPi national conferences along with many local and regional conclaves and student meetings. The AEPi fraternity's international board was comprised of all adults, plus two student members. My senior year, one of those two lone students who were chosen from all the student members all over the world was me! My responsibilities were huge, as I had a vote on the board, and my vote represented all the student members of the AEPi fraternity. I did not take these responsibilities lightly, and I made sure I heard from as many students as possible before I cast my vote. We voted on budgets and policy and on many other things that affected not only current undergrad members but also those who would come after us.

During my term, I traveled to several national meetings and discussed topical issues with the adult members of the board. At all times I was taken seriously and respected; not once did Tourette syndrome become an issue or turn into a problem. I was very encouraged by this and hoped that the trend would continue when I began searching for my first teaching job the next summer.

Not wanting to leave the job search until the last minute, I used winter break to drive to Atlanta and check out possible teaching positions. I met with a few principals, made lots of contacts, and basically put together a game plan for the following summer. I left Atlanta that winter with peace of mind. I knew I was coming back.

In the spring of 1996, I graduated cum laude from Bradley University. It was the day I had always hoped for and sometimes thought would never arrive. I was now officially ready to teach! It had been a long, winding road leading to this moment, and I was thrilled to be able to share my graduation with so many of the important people in my life. In addition to my immediate family—Mom, Dad, Jeff, and my stepmother, Diane—also able to attend were my Big Brother, Steve Mathes, his wife, Julie, and their younger son, Joey. I was especially pleased that Steve and his family made the drive. We had kept in touch throughout my college years, and it meant a lot to me that they were there. And, throughout my high school and college years, Dad had begun to change his thinking about Tourette's and about me. We had a ways to go, but we were headed in the right direction.

The graduation was bittersweet, as I was leaving so many good friends, but I was excited about the opportunities that lay ahead. If the upcoming move to Atlanta didn't work out, I knew I could always go back to St. Louis, but I was willing to take a chance on my chosen southern city. That chance ended up paying off, but not without a lot of heartbreak first.

9

BARKING UP THE WRONG TREES

I WAS FRESH OUT OF COLLEGE in June of 1996 when I packed up the old Volvo once again for a drive to Atlanta. I was finally going to do the job search that would begin my life as a teacher. The long drive through Illinois, Kentucky, and Tennessee gave me a lot of time to think about where I might teach. What school? What grade?

I had no expectations of anything being handed to me, but I wasn't particularly worried about finding a job, either. My stint as a student teacher had gone so well that I had come away from it assured that my dream of leading a classroom was a true calling. I knew that some of my confidence came from spending the previous four years with people I knew and liked—and people who liked me and who understood about my tics. A lot of potential social difficulties can be avoided in an atmosphere like that. But I had grown so much as a person during my college years that I felt sure I could make people outside my little world understand Tourette's, too. And so it was easy to drive along reveling in my dream of standing in front of a class of children eager to hear what we were all going to do that day. I couldn't wait to launch into the ongoing daily battle for their attention, for their learning, and for their respect.

Before I left St. Louis, I happened to hear that the roommate of one of my friends in Atlanta was going to be away for the summer and needed to sublet in order to keep his lease. I jumped at the chance to move in and spend the summer months finding my first full-time teaching job.

In the meantime, during the early part of the summer I had the opportunity to return to Camp Alterman, this time as a unit head—a counselor with supervisory responsibilities.

Leslie Jaslow, my unit head from the previous summer, said she was really glad to see me back. "You have a wonderful relationship with each and every kid," she told me. "You never sit around while the kids play; you join in all the games and never take a break, and the parents love you. I'm proud to have you on my staff."

These were wonderful words, and I would draw strength from them later in the summer. From my perspective, the camp job was a stroke of luck, as I could schedule my job interviews around my duties at camp.

Throughout those months, I did what every determined person does when looking for meaningful work—every time I ran into a friend or acquaintance, I asked for leads on teaching jobs. And just in case an interview opportunity popped up at the last moment, I kept my good navy pin-striped suit hanging in my car, along with the appropriate shirt, tie, and shoes.

✳ ✳ ✳

In most schools within the gigantic Atlanta school system, the formal application process works like this: you put in an application with the human resources office, then wait for school principals to call you for an interview. I hated the idea of waiting for the right school to "find" me, but that was the process. I applied at all the major school districts to increase my chances of getting calls. Then I waited the same long, painful wait known by everyone who has ever sweated their way through a job search, sitting by the phone for a call. Whoever first said "time drags" was probably waiting to hear about a job.

When the first call finally came, it was from a recruiter for one of the largest and most diverse school districts in Atlanta. The woman said they liked my application and wanted to meet me. This was exciting! Wearing my navy pin-striped suit, the shirt, the tie, and the shoes, I charged into the human resources office at the appointed time and eagerly handed over my résumé. The recruiter asked me a lot of questions, and because of other interviews I'd done in the past, I had most of the answers memorized.

"What is your philosophy of teaching?"

I was prepared for that one. "My philosophy of education is to . . . RAH . . . allow students a chance to succeed by WOOP providing hands-on experiences . . ." I talked about how important it is to communicate with parents, to give children choices in the classroom, and to offer them a voice in their own learning. I explained that I wouldn't let race, income, ethnicity, language difficulties, or anything else interfere with teaching those children. I felt it was my responsibility to use every available resource to be certain that each child learned at the appropriate level.

The recruiter asked how I would maintain discipline. I told her about a flip-card chart I used to hold children accountable for their behavior. Each week I would send a report home to parents, letting them know how their child was doing in terms of both academics and behavior.

I described my work as a camp counselor, told the recruiter about my colleagues naming me Counselor of the Year, and let her know how much the honor meant to me.

We both knew that sooner or later the subject of Tourette's had to come up—there was no way to hide the fact that I had TS, and I wanted to be open about it anyway. By law, I did not have to disclose my Tourette's or even talk about it. By law, prospective employers were not supposed to bring it up, but if I initiated the discussion it was all right to address the issue.

Finally, I felt ready to open the topic. I explained that my technique for informing students about my condition was to give them a frank description of it as a neurological disorder with unavoidable tics that were like sneezes—when you have to, you have to. I also let the recruiter know that the kids were allowed to ask questions about it at any time. She asked how the children reacted to Tourette's in general, and I assured her that once they got used to it, they were unfazed. She seemed to absorb the Tourette's stuff more intensely than my views on discipline and teaching. As the interview drew to a close, I felt exhilarated. I was learning how to meet job interview challenges and to anticipate the answers that I needed to have prepared.

Throughout the rest of the session, the interviewer smiled and nodded as if I were playing Trivial Pursuit and getting every question right. It was only toward the end that her voice took on a slightly more subdued tone.

"I think it might be hard for you to find a job, Brad," she said. "People just aren't used to the possibility that a successful teacher would have Tourette syndrome. As if teaching isn't difficult enough for anyone . . ."

Deep down, I'd expected to hear someone say something like this. It's the attitude that every person with a disability dreads encountering—when someone just isn't willing to give us a chance. Even after so many years of dealing with strangers' reactions, the interviewer's words still cut me wide open. I knew I could work with children, and I'd been able to prove it many times over. But how could I convince a stranger who hadn't seen me teach that Tourette's wouldn't get in the way?

I tried the direct approach: "I just want a chance to prove to principals that I can do the job."

She smiled and nodded. "Best of luck, Brad," she said. Then she signed me up to interview with principals from three different schools. Maybe she couldn't find it in herself to hold out any hope, but at least she had agreed to let me try the interview process. That was enough . . . for now. I went home and updated my portfolio, then began to obsess in the process of running every possible question and answer through my mind.

The interview appointments with all three principals turned out to be on the same day, which was a little intense but was the best way to do it while still showing up for my duties at camp. So I went to work as usual, with my suit in the car, and put in a few hours being a camp counselor before leaving early for the interviews.

Atlanta is a huge city, so my first challenge was to navigate the complex highway system, chance the unpredictable traffic, and still be on time. After I left camp, I had to take I-285, one of Atlanta's legendary frightening and perplexing highways. It was impossible not to be terrified of getting lost and missing the interview. I remembered a story about a Braves baseball player who missed his first game because he kept going round and round on I-285, looping endlessly around the city. Hopefully the same would not happen to me.

My luck held. I found the right exit, pulled into a McDonald's, and used the restroom to change into my suit. All I needed was an old-time phone booth, and I would have felt like Clark Kent getting into his Superman costume. When I came out, an elderly lady even looked at me curiously and asked, "Were you in there with your twin, or did you change clothes?"

My feats weren't quite as astounding as Superman's, but I felt a lot like him as I arrived at the elementary school on time with my résumé in hand. It was really happening. I was finally getting a chance to start my teaching career.

I interviewed first with a principal who needed teachers for either the fourth or the fifth grade. The principal wouldn't be absolutely sure about the grade assignment until closer to the start of the school year. She told me about her school, emphasizing that her teachers had to work with a diverse population. I assured her that that would not be a problem. Some of my own student teaching had been carried out at a magnet school in inner-city Peoria. Yes, the cultural atmosphere was different, but kids are kids; they all need a positive and supportive learning environment, and they do best under a disciplinary program that involves self-enforcement with reasonable consequences.

Naturally, I brought up Tourette syndrome, and when I launched into my explanation, the principal leaned forward and listened intently. I even showed her the articles about me that had run in the *Peoria Journal Star*. It felt great to have them, because good newspaper articles written by someone else reflect on you much more positively than you yourself saying how great you are. She looked the articles over, then smiled and thanked me for coming in, saying she'd call me when she had made a decision. I left without being able to judge her response. Her professional demeanor was pleasant but completely opaque. All I knew for sure was that I had one down and two to go.

The second principal was older, a seasoned administrator who said she wanted to see more men in elementary school classrooms because so many children were growing up in single-mother homes. She knew they needed all the positive male role models they could get. She smiled the whole time we talked.

"I see that you have Tourette syndrome, and that you've been very successful with it," she said while she flipped through the newspaper articles in my portfolio.

It was wonderful to hear her recognition. "I've been fortunate," I said. "WOOP, woop, woop, many people with Tourette's don't graduate from college."

She seemed to know more about Tourette's than most people, and didn't indicate that she thought it would prevent me from teaching. Like the previous principal, she said she'd be in touch once she had made a decision. Even though she was friendlier than the first principal, once again I found her professional polish to be so smooth that I had no idea what she actually thought.

The principal at the final interview was a younger woman, and she stood and greeted me like an old friend. I got the definite impression that someone had forewarned her about the noises I made, so I decided to test the situation by not bringing up Tourette's. It would be interesting to find out what an interview was like when Tourette syndrome wasn't part of the conversation.

Big mistake.

Legally, she was not supposed to bring up the topic. But as the interview dragged on, the "elephant in the room" grew bigger and bigger, and I began to regret not talking about Tourette's. By going so long without mentioning it, I allowed the topic to feel all the more awkward. The interview ended without TS ever being mentioned, and I left feeling empty and disappointed in myself. I felt as if I'd been hiding my condition—as if I were ashamed of myself—when actually Tourette's is so much a part of who I am and what I have accomplished that to keep it a secret is to withhold a giant piece of myself from the world. By now, I'd accepted Tourette syndrome as a constant companion—a companion I could no longer imagine being without.

I decided that if I went to future interviews, I would be up front about Tourette's. Then it would be out in the open—and if I did get the job, there wouldn't be any surprises. I've heard about job applicants with Tourette syndrome who successfully keep their noises and twitches in check for the interview, only to show up for the job and quickly find themselves with a lot of explaining to do. I didn't want to teach anywhere where Tourette's made people uncomfortable or where the principal was unable or unwilling to create an environment in which people's differences were accepted.

My day ended with the general feeling that on the first two interviews, everything had gone as well as possible. But I had no idea what the principals were looking for or how many prospective teachers they were interviewing.

Since there were no guarantees, I continued job hunting while I waited to hear from the principals. But at this point, about midway through the summer, the stress was starting to build—in the way that anyone who's ever struggled to find work can understand. I had a strong urge to spend some serious relaxation time in an environment where the apparent limitations of Tourette syndrome wouldn't be right in my face.

And so it was a perfect time to step back from the grim routine of looking for work and enjoy the fact that within the span of just a few weeks, the whole world seemed to have shown up in Atlanta for the Summer Olympics. Everyone was talking about what events they were going to see. Jeff flew in from St. Louis and my dad managed to score tickets to one of the most sought-after events—the women's gymnastics competition. It seemed like a good idea. How much trouble can a guy get into for spontaneous shouting at an Olympic sporting event? I felt so safe about the situation that we also brought along two friends from St. Louis.

The Georgia Dome was jammed with spectators—every single seat was occupied. We were all talking and catching up as we made our way to our aisle and crammed into our seats. We were sitting up so high that I could barely distinguish the tiny American gymnasts from those from other countries.

As soon as we sat down, I started barking. My friends and my brother were unfazed. They hardly noticed anymore. But the people around us sure noticed. Every time I let out a noise, men and women of all ages turned and glared at me. The more I yipped and yelped, the more aggravated the people in front of us became.

One woman shushed me. I tried to explain about Tourette's, but she whipped around, shaking her head. Then a man stood up and stomped over to a nearby security guard. I watched his face contort while he told the security guard about all the "rude noises" I was making. He pointed to me, and he pointed to his ticket. It was easy to see his point—seats at Olympic events weren't cheap. Each of our tickets had a face value of about eighty-five dollars.

The security guard relayed the story to a volunteer, who came over to talk to us.

"He can't help it," Jeff explained. "He has Tourette syndrome. Do you know what that is?"

"Isn't that where you make noises all the time and sometimes you curse?" the volunteer asked.

"No," I said. "That kind of Tourette syndrome is very rare. I don't curse; I just make noises and jerk my head around."

As if on cue, I emitted a loud "Wah!"

The volunteer had no idea what to do. People were complaining and it was her job to make everyone happy. The competition was about to start and she needed a quick solution.

"I'm afraid if you don't quiet down, we're going to have to ask you to sit somewhere else," she said.

"He can't help it," Jeff repeated.

The volunteer looked stumped. "Let me go talk to some people, and I'll be right back, okay?"

She left, and we tried to enjoy the event, but by now we were all feeling tense. Jeff talked about how I had as much right to be there as the guy who had reported me to security. Our friends agreed. We talked about what we would do if the volunteer tried to make us move. We agreed on principle that it was wrong. But, as Jeff said, "It's not like our seats could be any worse." I just wanted to watch the competition and forget about the people sitting around me, but it seemed like my internal companion had other plans for all of us.

"Wah!"

By now, everyone within earshot was following our conversation. They didn't look at me when I made noises, but I could feel the tension. Remember, stress just makes Tourette's worse. Pretty soon, I saw the volunteer marching up the steps. Jeff walked down to her, and the two met with some official-looking people to talk about the situation.

A few minutes later, Jeff motioned all of us to follow him and the volunteer. Jeff had been through many scenes like this before; he knew what to do and I trusted his judgment, but I couldn't really believe this. Was Jeff agreeing that we would let ourselves be kicked out? This wasn't some hushed theater event or classical concert—it was an athletic competition. Despite my concerns, we all walked down the steps, lower and lower, until we were almost right on the floor with the athletes.

Then the volunteer stopped and pointed out four seats to us—four really great seats!

"Well, Brad, how's this?" she asked, smiling at us like a co-conspirator. She had just helped us to beat the intolerance of the complainers by granting their wish to see us moved. But these seats were far better than the others—instead of the eighty-five dollar seats, we were now sitting in the *two hundred* eighty-five dollar seats and were only about twenty-five rows from the floor. I wanted to hug her but had to settle for thanking her profusely. After she left, as we sank into our newer, better, far more comfortable seats, I couldn't keep the grin off of my face. Sometimes, in unexpected ways, Tourette's allows me glimpses of how a total stranger will feel empathy and make courageous decisions on another person's behalf. I even managed to get a laugh out of Jeff and our friends by wisecracking, "As you can see, there are advantages to having Tourette's. Enjoy the view!" We all gave each other high fives.

So the Olympics helped put me in a good mood, even though my job search was stalled and it was getting later in the summer. A nice day at a sporting event doesn't change the reality of things. I knew most principals had already hired their new teachers. So far, I'd successfully refused to let myself get discouraged, but that hill was getting harder and harder to climb every day. Everyone kept reminding me how hard it is to land your first job out of college. I always smiled and said that I was sure something would turn up soon.

For a long time, I believed it.

✳ ✳ ✳

I was still getting by with my work at Camp Alterman when I got a call from a principal who wanted to interview me later that same day. This would be approximately my eighteenth interview.

"Sure," I said, thankful I was still keeping the suit hanging in my car. I drove out of camp and found a nearby church parking lot where I could change clothes.

By the time I pulled up to the school I was already running through the usual interview questions in my head. How will you work with slow readers? How will you communicate with parents? At this point, I knew the routine so well that the answers spilled out of me on command. Even so, there were now only a few weeks until the school year began, and I still wasn't any closer to landing my first teaching job.

I always drove to each interview with the air conditioner on full blast, hoping to keep from showing up looking rumpled. Mid-August in Georgia can be stifling. Still, no matter how hard I tried to remind myself of the importance of appearing relaxed, I knew that desperation is hard to camouflage.

When I arrived for the interview, my tics were especially rough. As I turned off the ignition, I chomped down hard, and from deep in my diaphragm came a loud "Fa . . . fa!"

I kept extra pens in the car, as biting on a pen sometimes helps to settle my nerves. So I pulled out a green plastic pen and bit down on the cap. It seemed to help a little and the vocal tics took a pause. There wasn't any more preparation that could be done. Ready or not, it was time to go inside.

From the moment I entered the building, I realized this school felt different from the others. My first clue was that the hallway was dimly lit. Also, in the summer, schools typically smell of cleaning solvents and fresh paint, but here there was a musty odor. It generally smelled of neglect.

"May I help you?" The secretary smiled at me as I walked to the front desk. She could see I was there for an interview, wearing my winter blue suit in the middle of summer and toting a portfolio bulging with certificates, awards, and newspaper articles.

"Hi. I'm Brad Cohen," I said in my most confident, upbeat voice. "I have an eleven o'clock appointment with the principal."

She asked me to take a seat, but as soon as I sat down I knew it was only a matter of time before my everpresent companion would start to act up. And while I could temporarily keep the barking, yipping, and chomping at bay by physically struggling to stifle the tics, by suppressing them while I waited for the interview, there was a real risk that they would explode out of me at some point during my conversation with the principal.

The first yip slipped out as I squirmed in the hard chair, trying to get comfortable. The secretary flinched. She looked around and up at the ceiling, trying to find the source of the noise. At this point, she didn't even think to look at me. I decided not to take the time to speak up and explain, and continued running interview questions and answers through my head.

What all the interviews needed to boil down to, I figured, was my belief that every child can learn. No matter what other questions the different principals asked, I felt sure that this assurance was what they wanted to hear. Each child can learn—must learn—for the child's own sake. If I were in these principals' shoes, interviewing prospective teachers, I know this is the kind of attitude and work ethic I'd be looking for. While I was doing all this thinking and still waiting to go into the principal's office, my neck suddenly jerked to one side, whipping the muscles so hard that the stiff collar on my dress shirt cut into my skin.

"Rah . . . rah, RAH!"

It burst out of me with such force that my torso jerked forward.

The secretary jumped from her seat as if a rock had just crashed through the window. Her eyes darted around the room, then settled on me—they were open wide. She looked as if she were staring down a ghost.

I still didn't say anything. The giant wall clock showed almost eleven fifteen. Where was this guy? The waiting was just making me more agitated, setting the stage for an even more spectacular introduction to the various facets of Tourette syndrome.

"Wah!"

My mouth opened as wide as it possibly could, and my neck jerked back and snapped forward. This time the secretary looked right at me, and I locked eyes with hers.

"I can't help it," was all I could say.

There wasn't time for more than that—a tall figure finally appeared in the doorway. "You must be Mr. Cohen."

I got up and hustled toward the principal, glad to get away from the secretary's stare. For the sake of my own self-confidence, I didn't need to dwell on what she must have thought of me. I could feel her stare as we left, but I didn't want to think about her and psych myself out, so I focused on the principal.

He was a thin man, sharply dressed, and although he was older than many other principals, he looked to be in good physical shape. When he extended his hand, I reached out expecting a firm, athletic grip, but his hand was limp against mine. It felt symbolic, somehow, of how different this school was from the others, even though I tried to force any negative thoughts from my mind. There was no way I could be picky about a job. Not this late in the summer.

Even so, most new teachers understand that it's especially important to get a good principal with your first teaching job. An elementary school is like a small town, and the principal is the mayor. The principal's position is a job that requires political savvy as well as strong leadership. That strength of leadership will ultimately have a direct impact on the teacher's ability to do his or her best in the classroom day after day. The importance of the principal's role makes a questionable proposition out of simply grabbing a teaching job just because it is offered. An uninvolved or uninspired principal may have little or no concern for the very things a new teacher will need most to succeed in the position.

Nevertheless, I willingly followed along when this tardy, limp-handed man in the musty-smelling building asked me to come back to his office. I wanted to see his work domain and how he decorated the room. After visiting so many principals' offices over the summer, I'd come to think that the quality of the office decor bore some correlation to the quality of the school itself.

His office jarred me when I walked in. I felt as if I had left school and entered church. The walls were covered with plaques bearing religious expressions and biblical verses. There were pictures of angels, and one of Jesus. A sign said, "SCHOOL RULES FROM 1812," and the first rule was "START EACH DAY WITH A PRAYER."

"Please, have a seat," he quietly began.

He told me about his school, and about the kids. "If it weren't summer, the kids would be here right now running through the halls and acting wild. These kids are tough. They need discipline. Let me just be frank about this—it's hard to work here. This is a school where teachers are expected to put in long hours."

"I'm all for that," I said. "I anticipate working hard."

My shirt collar was suddenly tight around my neck, and I could feel sweat forming on my temples. Without warning, my neck jerked back and forth, and I let out a lone, irrepressible "Wah!"

I knew I was going to bring up Tourette's, as I'd resolved always to do, but this forced the topic to the forefront. However—unbelievably—the man continued talking about his school as if he hadn't noticed the noise. I wondered if he was attempting to be tactful. His voice remained congenial, even though he spoke with authority. He seemed to have done this interview process a lot and to have a clear idea of what he was looking for. He told me there was an opening in fifth grade, which sounded promising since I'd already worked with fifth-graders as a student teacher. He also needed someone to teach math. I told him that would be fine, too.

His eyes took me in. "Tell me your philosophy of education."

I began my story, which by this time I could tell in my sleep, touching on the importance of hands-on activities instead of relying upon the use of mandatory worksheets as "baby-sitters." I stressed my opinion that a teacher needs to work closely with parents. I told him about my flip-chart reward system, and the need for weekly notes to parents.

He picked up my résumé.

"I see you graduated from Bradley University. That's a small college, isn't it?"

"Yes, it is."

"A small Catholic college, right? In the Boston area?"

"Well, no," I began evenly, trying not to lean too hard on his mistakes. "Actually it isn't a Catholic college. And it's located in Illinois. Peoria."

It was as if I hadn't said a word. "A Catholic college, isn't it?" he repeated.

"No, sir. The school isn't Catholic." By now I had to wonder. Why would he think I would either lie about that or somehow did not know the correct answer?

He continued to insist that Bradley University was in Boston and was a Catholic school, and his persistence was just irritating enough that I abandoned common sense and repeatedly corrected him, despite my need for the job. Right about the time that I was ready to give up on the whole interview, he conceded that perhaps he was thinking of another school.

"Brad," he finally said, "I see you have Tourette syndrome. I don't know too much about that. Tell me about it."

At last! It was out. He seemed eager to learn, and I was relieved to see that he wasn't going to try to ignore my tics and avoid the discussion.

"It's a neurological disorder," I began. "It causes my body to twitch and to make noises that I can't control. The tics are worse when I'm nervous, but once I relax, they quiet down. Children are curious about Tourette's, but once I explain it to them, they are fine with it. I tell them that it's like having the hiccups. Sometimes I compare it to the need to sneeze. They relate to that."

When I finished, he leaned forward and issued his verdict. "To tell you the truth, Brad," he said, then paused as if he didn't know quite how to proceed, "I can't see you as a teacher. I feel like Tourette syndrome would get in the way. I just don't know how you could teach."

"Excuse me?" I had to mentally rewind what he'd just said: *I can't see you as a teacher.*

He shook his head. "Brad—they'd laugh at you all day long. They wouldn't be able to concentrate or do their work. In all my years as an educator, I've known a lot of teachers—and I have never met one with Tourette syndrome."

I felt my cheeks get hot. And of course at this worst possible of moments, I released a piercing yip and my neck jerked to one side, once again hitting my shirt collar so hard the skin on my neck was rubbed raw.

He didn't flinch. There was no need to; he was watching me "prove" that he was right.

"I assure you, sir, that I *can* teach. In fact, I think I'm a better teacher because I have battled to overcome this disability.

I was a student teacher and I was very successful. Tourette's wasn't the problem that you say it is. In fact, it wasn't a problem at all."

He remained silent. I imagined him conjuring up a vision of me in the classroom, making noises in front of twenty-five fifth-graders. He leaned closer. "The kids I'm dealing with at this school . . . in this community . . . they would beat you up if you made noises like that all day. You wouldn't be safe here. Do you understand what I'm telling you?"

I started to count backward from ten. Even though this was clearly not a school where I wanted to work, I needed a job so badly that I didn't want to burn any bridges. It seemed obvious that I couldn't persuade this man to hire me, given his opinions about people with Tourette syndrome.

He summed up his feelings this way: "If you want to teach, you need to refrain from making noises during class time."

I stood up and brushed off my jacket. "Thank you for the interview."

He looked confused, like I was a guest at his home departing early. "You're leaving?"

"I don't think this is the teaching position for me," I said, trying to stay calm and upbeat. "But again, thank you for the interview. I'll take my portfolio and not ask for any more of your time."

I reached for my portfolio, and he released it without objection. In my wallet, I had my folded piece of paper with highlights of the Americans with Disabilities Act printed on it. Part of me wanted to pull the paper out and recite from it, the way I sometimes did in movie theaters when managers tried to throw me out. Instead, I walked out of his office, through the reception area, and past the secretary, who, it is safe to say, was most certainly relieved to see the barking man in the dark suit depart the premises.

Once I got to my car, I gripped the steering wheel, breathing hard. Even though I can maintain my dignity in a situation like that, the fallout with tics and twitches is about as bad as you would imagine it to be. The disappointment was overwhelming, and I started in on the self-consolation routine that was becoming as much of a constant companion as the Tourette's itself. There would be other schools. There would be other chances.

I reminded myself that it would be a nightmare to work at a place like that anyway. Even so, I hated the idea of just walking away as if everything were okay. The man had discriminated against me in a stupid and stereotyped way, denying me the chance to earn an honest living. He had broken the law. Furthermore, he was just the kind of person who would have to have somebody stand their ground with him before he would ever open his eyes. In the past, I had always stood my ground as much as possible when it came to defending my rights. I could have sued—should have sued—but after this encounter, it didn't seem worth the effort.

Just as I was about to start the car, I felt a sharp, burning pain in my neck. I loosened my tie and unbuttoned my dress shirt, then pulled down the rearview mirror so I could see what was going on. Underneath my shirt collar, my skin was bleeding from all the neck twitching.

I couldn't get away from that school fast enough. I turned the key in the ignition and pulled out of the parking lot, but by the time I found the main road that would lead me home, I couldn't see. Tears blurred my vision. I pulled over to the side of the road and dropped my forehead into my hands.

It's over, I thought. No principal will ever look past my disability. It seemed clear that Tourette's had finally gotten the better of me for real. It had stopped me from doing the thing I had always wanted most to do: teach kids and let them find joy in learning. For a while I just sat there, watching cars whiz by.

By this point in the deepening summer, a thought that I'd been fighting for months was becoming more and more insistent. What if no one will hire me because I have Tourette's? How many other principals are going to see me as merely a victim of Tourette syndrome instead of an educated and qualified teacher?

Then I breathed deeply and felt my lungs fill with air. I told myself to erase any thought of giving up. Plenty of doors had been slammed in my face before, and things somehow always managed to work out.

One thing at a time. Later, at home, I could figure out what to do next about finding a teaching job. For now, I just needed to drive.

✳ ✳ ✳

When the summer drew to a close, my camp job ran out and, with no money coming in, I was officially unemployed. I still went to interviews, but my eyes had been opened to the pitying way in which some people insisted upon viewing me. My confidence was eroding.

Whenever I spoke on the phone with my parents, they asked how the job search was going, and the question made me cringe.

"It's coming along," was my standard reply.

That was enough information for my father, but my mother wasn't buying it. "You know, Brad, you could come back to St. Louis," she ventured one day.

No sane parent wants to see his or her child crawling back home after a failed job search—my father especially had no interest in that—but Mom didn't hesitate to hold out the opportunity to me if that was what I needed. I thanked her but emphasized that I wasn't quitting.

What she didn't understand was that I personally could absolutely not use Tourette's as an excuse. Even if I believed that it was the reason I couldn't get a job—even if I knew for a fact that it was the reason I wasn't being hired—I couldn't let myself say those words out loud. That would give the reality of it too much weight.

By that point, my quest to become a teacher was completely linked to my drive for survival. If I was going to exist with any degree of dignity and independence, then I had no choice but to prove that Tourette syndrome would never get the best of me.

It became clear to me then: if I were to let go of my determination, I wouldn't have any direction left. Nor would I have any way to cope with not having a worthwhile purpose in life. If I quit now, I would be agreeing with everyone who had been telling me all summer that I was barking up the wrong trees. I had to decide whether it was the kind of tree in general—

meaning my chosen career—that was wrong, or whether it was the location of the trees individually—meaning that I had not yet found the right school. Because I felt so strongly about being a teacher, I decided I had not yet found the right school. I'd keep barking. I was not quitting.

10

Dire ... Ire ... Mire ... Hire

IN THE MIDDLE OF MY JOB SEARCH, I moved into a new apartment with Jordan Hirschfield, a friend from St. Louis (and one of my roommates from the previous summer). I'd scouted the apartment while still working at Camp Alterman and I loved it on first sight. Located in a brand-new gated complex in a busy area of Atlanta that was perfect for young, single professionals, it was exactly the apartment I had envisioned for myself after college—we each had our own bedroom, with TV and stereo equipment in the den. As soon as we moved in, we made a joint purchase of a gas grill just like the ones people had back in St. Louis. The only missing ingredient was that little thing called a job.

All summer now, I had been doing the job hunter's daily hustle, sending out as many résumés with cover letters as I could find people to send them to. Some had resulted in interviews, but each of those later resulted in rejection letters. Each day I hurried out to the mailbox. If one of the envelopes I pulled out was from a school I'd interviewed at, then I made it an exercise in self-restraint not to rip it open right there on the spot. Instead I waited until I got inside. Even then, before opening the envelope I gave myself a pep talk: "If it's another rejection, I'll just keep interviewing. I'll get a job soon. I won't panic."

Sometimes while I stared at the sealed envelope I drifted into a brief fantasy about how I would react if I got the job. I'd imagine the joy of knowing I had finally reached my goal of being a teacher. I'd visualize the kids and my desk, the teacher's lounge, and the crowded halls. But the letters were all using different words that said the same thing: they would not be extending an offer, but thanks for the interest. Even though I realized they were rejecting Tourette's and not me, the words were still hard to take. Tourette's was such a big part of me that you didn't get the rest of me without the Tourette's.

Before too long, the drumbeat of serial rejection began to take its toll, and I began to use more and more energy fighting panic. Even though I worked every contact I could possibly find, the hiring season was ending and interviews were drying up. Time was running out. I queried various school district administrators, but they told me to just wait for a call, wait for more openings to come available. The days began melting into an endless blur of *CHiPs* reruns, and as each new day came it was harder and harder to get off the couch.

Meanwhile, my constant companion was very present. Old tics I hadn't seen since junior high reemerged as if they'd never left. I chomped my teeth together violently as my head twitched from side to side. My head sometimes shook so hard that Jordan said it looked like it might fly off. Sometimes I slammed my head back with such force that my neck was in a constant state of soreness, and the pain became more intense with every jerk and tic.

My usual tics were also coming faster and louder, wearing out my body and sapping my strength. I knew it was important to keep my spirits up throughout the job search process, but the overwhelming physical exhaustion caused by the tics just didn't leave me with any resources to meet the task. Despite my determination to remain positive, I began sliding backward.

When I first moved to Atlanta, I had a very active social life and spent most of my free time with friends. We went out a few nights a week. Now I rarely left the apartment. It was so much easier to just stay home and not have to answer a lot of depressing questions about how the ol' job hunt was going. Besides, my tics were never as bad at home as they were out in public, and I needed as much time away from them as I could get.

By late August I was as discouraged as I had ever been. Diane, my stepmother, visited me in my new apartment and tried to give me some confidence. I tried to take Diane's encouragement—and the kind words of all my friends—to heart, but it was tough. Recently she recalled the situation: "No one was willing to risk hiring a teacher with Tourette syndrome, and Brad was so discouraged. Despite the glowing recommendations he presented, he kept having doors close in his face."

Later, after Diane had left and I was alone with my thoughts again, I decided I had to come up with some sort of plan. I realized that I might need to consider starting off as a substitute teacher, just to get into the schools. That way, at least people would see what I could do in a classroom. But then I thought some more. Would the barrier to that route be any different? If the people who did the hiring actually believed I wouldn't be fit as a full-time teacher, would they be any more inclined to give me access to the same students, just because I was dubbed a "substitute" teacher instead?

No matter how I reasoned it out, the same answer kept coming back: I am a teacher. I was born for this. I have to teach. I am not going to let anything stop me.

The late Joseph Campbell, a great teacher and mythologist, described a phenomenon that is often found in stories of life-or-death struggles. It is the moment when the hero finds himself or herself inside what Campbell called the "Innermost Cave." The Innermost Cave is that point in a long and arduous journey or battle when all the hero's resources are exhausted. Even the inner resources of self-confidence become useless. Inside this Innermost Cave, the hero will either fall into despair and be defeated, and the journey will end, or he or she will spontaneously develop some new ability and survive to fight another day.

I was deep inside my Innermost Cave, and I knew it was time for me to take a giant and aggressive leap forward in my social marketing skills. Whether or not it felt natural for me to sell myself to strangers, I had to do it and do it better than I ever had before. And to be successful at that, I needed to make some sort of new push unlike anything I'd done so far—because somehow I had to find a principal who was willing to take a chance on hiring me. That was all there was to it.

I knew my principal was out there. I just hadn't found him or her yet.

The next morning I got up especially early. My new resolve had filled me with an inordinate amount of energy. Instead of moving from the bed to the couch and making another rerun marathon out of the day—and instead of obsessing over my unemployment—I resolved to drive around and make impromptu visits to a new list of schools over the course of a single day. At each one, I would walk in smiling, greet anyone who would talk to me, introduce myself, and drop off as many résumés as I could. Despite my depressed state, I knew I could muster up enough energy for a plan like this if I made the entire effort in a single, long burn.

When it came time to saddle up for the day, I put on the old pin-striped suit, printed out a map of all the schools from the computer, then grabbed a stack of freshly printed résumés and took off. Inside the car, I cranked up the air and pointed the vents at my face, the usual routine in my quest to avoid looking sweaty in front of a future boss. This morning it felt especially right to appear at my best. The first stop on the long route was a large elementary school in a nice suburban area. I spoke with the secretary in the main office, who smiled and told me that the principal was unavailable. She gave me a second professional smile, took my résumé, and wished me luck. Strike one.

I got back in my car and looked on the map for the next school. As I've mentioned before, metro Atlanta is not an easy city for a newcomer to figure out. Many streets have the same name even though they are entirely different roads. There are over fifty streets called Peachtree-something. Many streets end abruptly and then inexplicably resume a half mile later. Other streets change names, sometimes every few blocks.

I couldn't help thinking about my mother's invitation to return to St. Louis, but I repeated to myself that it could never be an option. Over the years I had met too many people with Tourette's who had given up on their lives. Their plights made me determined never to let myself get to that point, because I strongly suspected that if I failed to break into the teaching profession now, then this same failure would set off a series of defeats that would eventually become my downfall. I was reminded once again of my initial experience with the Tourette syndrome support group meeting and the sad lives those people had all fallen into. The thought gave me enough resolve to finish my plan for the day.

In that cheerful frame of mind, I arrived at the next school on the list. Again I spoke with a secretary, gave her my résumé, and smiled back when she informed me that the principal was unavailable.

When I arrived home in the middle of the afternoon, I'd visited twenty schools. Who says manic outbursts aren't useful? Exhausted, I went inside, peeled off my suit, and chugged down a glass of water. What a day. Just as I was about to fall into bed for a nap, the phone rang. The man on the line asked if I was still looking for a teaching position.

"Yes, I am," I said, trying not to sound too eager.

"I'm Jim Ovbey," he went on. "I'm the principal at Mountain View Elementary. We were wondering if you could come in for an interview today."

Hmmm . . . Oh, let's see. Could I?

I remained heavy on the professionalism and light on the desperation while we set up an appointment for four thirty that afternoon. Then he handed the phone to the assistant principal, Hilarie Straka, and she gave me directions.

My heart was racing when I hung up. Handing out those résumés was a great idea, I thought. Even though I had not gone to that particular school, the school community was so well connected that résumés were floated around right and left, and names of likely candidates were exchanged like cheers at a sporting event. Someone I had seen earlier might even have put in a good word for me. I put my suit back on, grabbed my portfolio, and headed back into the summer heat and the rush-hour traffic.

What I didn't know then was that Jim Ovbey was more than a little concerned about the barking sounds I had made on the phone. I apparently was barking so loudly and so frequently that Jim had problems concentrating on our conversation.

"All the time I wondered what it would be like to have a man like Brad working with us," Jim said later. "Would we, and the children and their parents, be strong enough to work with him?"

At the time, Mountain View Elementary had six self-contained classes for children with learning disabilities.

"We had told those children time after time that they could do anything they wanted to do or be anything they wanted to be," Jim continued. "And, as Hilarie, my assistant principal, said, 'If we are going to talk the talk, then we'd better walk the walk.'"

All of this was unknown to me when I arrived at Mountain View, finding the school perched on a hill at a busy intersection. The school was in Cobb County, a suburban district that families moved into because of the strong reputation of the schools. On that afternoon, the parking lot was empty because it was a few days before teachers had to report. A week after that, the kids would arrive to begin the new school year.

From the outside, Mountain View didn't seem much different from many of the other elementary schools I had visited. It was square, brown, and unremarkable. But inside, I noticed that the office had a clean, crisp appearance. Despite the inexpensive wicker furniture, someone with a sense of style had given the space a nice decorator's touch. Classical music played softly in the hallway, and from somewhere came the soothing chirps of parakeets.

Then I met Jim and Hilarie, both casually dressed and waiting for me. As soon as we entered Jim's office, I felt more comfortable than I had at any of the other schools. They asked me a lot of the standard questions about teaching and about what kind of position I wanted.

Jim asked why, out of all the other choices I might have made, I wanted to be a teacher. Principals never failed to ask me this, and I always loved responding. Somehow, it made me stronger just to hear myself saying the words to someone else.

"I want to teach so I can be the teacher I never had," I said. "I want to be a RAH! supportive force in my students' lives. I . . . woop, woop! . . . believe that's the best way to help children learn and grow."

The questions kept coming, and the answers poured out of me. It felt great to speak of all these dreams with people who honestly seemed to be interested in hearing me. And I could tell by the way Jim and Hilarie both nodded their heads that they liked my responses. By the time Tourette's came up I felt completely at ease.

I told them about the many times I had explained Tourette's to children, and how they reacted. "I don't ever want Tourette's to be a . . . JA! ja, ja . . . topic that's off-limits," I told them. "I like to be open and honest, and if a question is too personal, WOOP, I just say it's too personal and move on."

Jim had been sitting behind his desk with his fingers laced behind his head. Now he leaned toward Hilarie and me and spoke in a solemn tone. "I hope this isn't too personal," he began.

I straightened in my chair and told him to fire away. I was expecting the worst.

"Do you make those noises in your sleep?"

Hilarie burst out laughing. So did I. I'd answered about a million questions that summer, but none of the other interviewers had asked this particular question. Jim said he was just curious, and I assured him it was a fair question.

"No, I don't make noises in my sleep," I said, "because I'm so relaxed."

The interview went on for more than two hours. At one point, Hilarie asked me if I liked Chinese food. When I said yes, though a bit surprised by that question, she laughed and said that when an interview was going well, she liked to break up the predictable questions with an unexpected one. She had three she chose among: (1) What is the best shopping day for sales? (2) What is T's? (3) Do you like Chinese food?

Well, I didn't know anything about shopping and wasn't familiar with T's, either, which I later learned was a local restaurant. But I liked Chinese food just fine, and the more time I spent at Mountain View, the more apparent it was to me that I liked this school a lot, along with the unique atmosphere that Jim and Hilarie had created.

The interview lasted long enough for Jim to see what I meant about not making noises in my sleep. The longer I stayed in his office, the fewer noises I made. None of my other interviews had lasted long enough for me to get so relaxed.

At the end of the interview, Jim and Hilarie both said they wanted me to meet with their fifth grade teachers, which was a very good sign. We made an appointment for a few days later.

"I knew from our interview that Brad was a very strong person—not overpowering, but a leader and someone the children would look up to," recalled Jim. "We felt confident that Brad would be a good teacher if given the opportunity. We just had to be sure we had a place for him."

I left feeling exhilarated; I knew there was really a chance this time! Even though the school year was on the verge of starting, it was still possible to get a late-entry teaching job. At Mountain View, Jim suspected that he might need to add a fifth grade teacher to accommodate the new families that moved to the district over the summer. The suburban communities of Atlanta were growing fast, with new homes appearing as quickly as construction crews could build them. School principals typically didn't know exactly how many students they would have when the school year started. That's why each year there was always a last-minute shuffling of teachers and a very few positions that came open late. I thought about all those new houses on cul-de-sacs and hoped fervently that there would be enough fifth-graders to warrant another class at Mountain View. Any size class would be fine. Any size class at all.

The day of the next interview came, and the meeting with the fifth grade teachers went very well, even though only three of them could make it. We all crowded around a little table in the school library while they passed my portfolio around. They noted that I had worked with fifth-graders as a student teacher, and that was good, but these people were classroom veterans. I have to admit that I was more than a little intimidated.

I called the school every few days, and Hilarie told me to be patient. I did a few more interviews in the meantime, but none went as smoothly as the one at Mountain View. By now, the school year had begun and I was really getting antsy. Patience was never my strong suit, and I worked hard to keep the impatience from turning into despair. I felt good about the interview at Mountain View, but I also tried not to dwell on the fact that no matter how good the interview felt, I was still very much in the ranks of the unemployed.

At home, my tics kept acting up. Yip. Jerk. Bark. Chomp. I debated whether I should waste time trying to substitute teach, or if I should look for a part-time job doing something else. But what else? Teaching is my passion; it's what I know how to do. Anything else would feel like a waste of time. I was so drained. When I wasn't stewing over my unemployment, I was worrying about what kind of excuse to give my folks the next time they called.

When friends called, I gave reasons why I couldn't go out. I said I was tired, which was true because of all the ticcing.

Often I fibbed and said I had other plans. Later, if one of those friends asked how my weekend had gone, I casually said those plans had fallen through. I really wanted to keep in touch with the friends I had made earlier in the summer, but I just couldn't bear to go out and field more questions about not having a job. I didn't want them to know how down I was. I didn't want them to know that Tourette's was keeping me from getting hired. I didn't want them to feel sorry for me.

Even though I had lived in Atlanta only a few months, I had made a lot of friends. I knew people from Camp Alterman, and I knew people from St. Louis who had moved to Atlanta. These friends introduced me to their friends, and my circle had expanded quickly. Everyone I met easily looked past the Tourette's and saw me as a person. So at least I knew that all the professional rejection wasn't from something in the local water supply. Why, then, couldn't these principals accept me the way other people in their town did? And why hadn't I heard from Mountain View?

Then one afternoon I got a call from Hilarie, who said they didn't need anyone for the fifth grade, but they might add a second grade teacher. She invited me to come in one more time and meet with the second grade staff. Second grade was fine with me, too. I certainly wasn't going to be picky, I thought, as I hurried over to meet them.

I found that the second grade teachers were all experienced, too, each with at least ten years in the classroom. But although they asked a lot of questions, they were essentially the same questions I'd been answering all summer. It was as if the summer itself had been a dress rehearsal for this very moment.

This was my twenty-fifth interview. I could predict in my sleep what question was coming next.

Again I got the feeling that the teachers were impressed, and I felt a spark of hope reigniting. There were four teachers this time. Two had serious attitudes, while the other two were more laid-back. They talked about all the things the teaching staff did as a team. They seemed like a fun, closely knit group.

When it was time for me to go, Jim and Hilarie took me aside and told me that the second grade teachers liked me. They needed to interview a few more candidates, but they would let me know by the end of the week. I drove out of the parking lot imagining myself as a Mountain View Elementary School teacher going home after a long day of classes. I sure wanted that vision to turn into a reality.

A few days passed—each day feeling like a week—and finally a woman from the school district's human resources department called. She asked if I would accept a job as a second grade teacher at Mountain View, and started to offer a little more information about the position.

She never got to the end of her spiel. I was hollering into the receiver, "I accept! I'll take it! Yes!" And with that, the long, intense search finally came to an end.

* * *

As soon as the job offer came in, my extra tics disappeared as quickly as they had come. I was happy about it because they were really wearing me out, but I was almost happier for my roommate, Jordan, because the extra pressure of the job search and the tics was affecting him, too.

"That summer, every school Brad interviewed with had a different excuse for why they couldn't hire him even though there were positions open," Jordan recalled. "Living with Brad really made me see how frustrating the ignorance of others can be. When the rejection letters started coming in, Brad's head started slamming backward really hard, and I worried that it would happen when he was driving and he'd knock himself out. But as soon as Mountain View had the sense to hire him, those tics stopped. The tics were just a negative reaction to the mindlessness of all the people who wouldn't give Brad the time of day."

For the rest of that day, my emotions ran the gamut from joy to exhilaration to disbelief and then back to joy. Even though I still had to show that I could deliver on my fervent desire to make the classroom a safe and fun place in which to learn—for all students—at last I would have the opportunity to try.

I felt like a mountain climber who has strained and struggled and finally—triumphantly—reaches base camp on Mt. Everest. A moment arrives when blunt, cold reality strikes: now that the wish to attempt the ascent has been granted, the would-be climber not only has to *actually climb* that daunting mountain—he has to make it back in one piece.

11

WE WON'T PLAY HIDE-AND-SEEK

WALKING INTO MOUNTAIN VIEW Elementary School as a teacher for the first time was a momentous occasion. Before I opened the door, I took a moment to look up at the United States flag blowing in the wind. I'd seen our flag so many times when I walked into other schools, but this time it had new meaning. It was the flag at the school where I was now a teacher.

My first day was a Thursday, and I had very little time to get my room ready and accomplish a lot of other preparatory tasks. My kids were already in classes with other teachers and would come to their new classroom for the first time the last hour of the day on Friday. They'd have the weekend to get used to the idea of a new classroom, and first thing Monday morning they would be all mine.

I didn't really have much for my classroom in the way of furniture or decorations—not even any desks. During my student teaching days, the cooperating teacher my senior year gave me the last week with her to make displays for the room I might eventually have. The things I made were intentionally pretty generic because I didn't know what grade I'd be teaching. I had Winnie the Pooh and Tigger items, pumpkins, a spaceman, a big "Writing Center" sign, a huge star chart, and a few other things. These were already laminated and ready to be hung. My cooperating teacher said that when I finally got my own class I wouldn't have time to make these things. She was definitely right about that. I had to work very quickly to get my room in order. Most teachers had a week to do what I needed to accomplish in just a day and a half. It was almost overwhelming; I had no idea how I'd get it all done.

While I was busy getting the room ready, the school administration was also preparing for my class. I had forms to send home to the parents of my new students, and information on my new students to read. I also had a meeting with Hilarie Straka to discuss the details of the children's own transition. Hilarie wrote a letter to the parents explaining that because of overcrowding in the second grade, their child would be switching classrooms and I would be the new teacher. She cautioned me that, initially, many of the parents would not be happy about the move because their children had been in school nearly three weeks and had made friends in their existing classrooms. But Hilarie and I both knew that children deal with change much better than most adults do. The kids would be fine.

"I knew Brad would get everyone past the Tourette's and win both the teachers and the parents over; they only had to meet him to see how exceptional he is," said Hilarie. "And he did bring everyone around. In just a matter of days Brad made people feel at ease."

What I didn't know at the time was that before they met me, some of the parents objected quite strongly to moving their child into my class.

"Brad was the new kid on the block, and the parents wanted to meet him before they acquiesced to the change," said Jim Ovbey. "My request to them was: you go up to Brad's room, meet him, and talk with him. After ten minutes you come back and tell me if he won't be good for your child. Only one parent still had concerns, which we honored. She later requested that her child be moved into Brad's class, but by then his class was filled and the opportunity for her child had passed."

I also prepared a letter to the parents to introduce myself and tell them a little about my philosophy and what they could expect. I was both excited and nervous about writing this letter. I had no clue whether I was doing it the right way. Only time would tell.

Later that first day, I went into each second grade classroom and introduced myself to all the students. Hilarie and I both thought it would make the transition easier if all the kids knew who I was, and it did. As I went to the different classrooms, the kids were all sitting on the floor, and when I walked in, their eyes opened wide, as if they were excited to see me. That was good, because I was very excited to see them. The kids didn't yet know which of them would be in my classroom, so they were all eager to learn about me.

Due to a combination of nervousness and excitement my tics were pretty bad, so we talked about Tourette syndrome right away. I told them I had a neurological disorder that made me make noises and tics I could not control.

"I was born with this . . . woop! . . . condition and right now JA! there's no medicine that can cure it," I said.

The looks on their faces were priceless. I told them that when I was awake I made noises more when I was nervous, in an uncomfortable situation, or when I got excited, but when I slept I didn't bark or tic at all. They understood right away.

A hand rose in the back of the room. A tall boy from the back of the class wanted to ask a question.

"Do you mean it's like blinking your eyes?" he asked. "My brain tells me to blink my eyes all day and I can't stop, but at night I go to sleep and don't blink."

That came out of a seven-year-old. The question triggered the floodgates.

"Do you go to movies?" one child asked.

"Yes, but sometimes I get kicked out and that makes me feel sad."

"Do you go to restaurants?" asked another.

I said that I did and that McDonald's was my favorite place to go.

"Does it hurt?" someone else asked.

"Sometimes the tics hurt, like when my neck jerks," I answered. "But the noises don't hurt at all."

"How many people have Tourette's?"

"Over one hundred thousand people have been diagnosed," I said, "but the actual number could be as high as one million because so many have not been diagnosed."

Another question came. "Do you know other people who have Tourette's?"

I told them how I have met a few, and that one, Jim Eisenreich, was even a major-league baseball player.

"Is it contagious?"

"No," I answered. "Tourette's is not . . . dra . . . DRA . . . contagious. You have to be woop! born with it." I added that the tics usually don't start until age seven or so.

One girl asked, "What can't you do with Tourette's?"

I asked what she meant.

"Like can you not eat or drink?"

I smiled and responded that, yes, I could eat and drink. But I also told them that they wouldn't be playing hide-and-seek with me, because they would always know where Mr. Cohen was. Mr. Cohen always loses at hide-and-seek. I mentioned that when I was growing up and I played hide-and-seek with my brother, he would always find me. All he had to do was say, "Brad, why aren't you making any noises?" Then I would think about the Tourette's and start to bark. He found me every time. I never was any good at that game, I told them. When all the kids laughed, I knew everything would be just fine.

* * *

After visiting all the second grade rooms, I still had a lot to do. I wanted to use the star chart to introduce my theme for the year: Reach for the Stars. But as soon as I got ready to hang it up, I noticed that I didn't have any tape. I also realized that I didn't have a stapler to staple papers together. Or any paper for the staples to go into. I didn't have any chalk, erasers, notebooks, or organizers. I had nothing.

As I began making a list of what I needed, all of a sudden one of the teachers walked in with a load of supplies. She shrugged off my thanks and said she thought I would need the things. I couldn't believe her timing. It was perfect.

A few minutes later, more teachers arrived, pulling a red wagon behind them. In the wagon were more supplies, games, and other much-needed things for my room. They said they had walked around the school with this "Welcome Wagon" and asked all the teachers to fill the wagon with items a new teacher might use or that they no longer wanted. This wagon was literally filled to the brim, practically overflowing with all kinds of things I would need to get started.

These teachers had gone out of their way to collect both necessities and niceties for me. I appreciated the supplies, but more than that, I was overwhelmed by the support that the teachers were showing by their actions. Then they surprised me once again, when they stayed after school to help me finish getting my room ready. I felt so honored. At first I said no, thank you. I knew they had more important things to do and families to attend to, but they insisted and began in earnest.

One donated item was a small, tremendously ugly lamp. One teacher painted it a pretty shade of blue for me. Another teacher helped hang things around the room. Another organized my supplies. Yet another fixed a coffee table that had broken legs. Before too long, I turned around to find that my room actually looked like a real second grade classroom.

Around seven o'clock, it was finally time to leave. There was still so much to do that I could have worked through the night, but I knew I needed to go home and get a good night's sleep. As I left the now quiet building, one of the custodians passed me and said, "Welcome to Mountain View. We're excited to have you here."

I couldn't believe the enthusiastic welcome I had received—from everyone! It was so comforting and comfortable. I loved this school!

As I walked to my car in the empty parking lot, I reflected on my first day. I knew in my heart that Mountain View was absolutely the right place for me. Although it had taken a desperately long time to get a job, I always knew I needed the right administration in order to be successful. Hilarie and Jim set the tone here, and the rest of the staff followed. They were all nice, and most welcomed me with open arms. I still couldn't quite believe that they were going to give me a chance to teach. Everyone here was able to see through the Tourette's and see me. It was a great feeling.

The next morning came early. Not only did I have to finish getting the classroom ready; I also needed to get my lesson plans together. And I didn't have a clue what I was supposed to teach.

* * *

There were 650 students at Mountain View Elementary. To form my class, each second grade teacher identified four or five kids from her class to move to my room. There had been four second grade classes. Mine would be the fifth. On Friday afternoon all my students headed to their new room. Since my room had no desks, they brought their own from their old classrooms. It was great. I heard the noise coming down the hall before anyone arrived. When I stuck my head out through the doorway, I saw a herd of seven-year-olds pushing their desks and chairs along the carpeted hallway toward me. It was the most wonderful sight I have ever seen! Once they arrived, they put their desks wherever they wanted. At the time, I didn't care where they were putting their desks. That was the least of my worries. I was trying to figure out how in the world I was going to remember all their names.

As the kids came in, some commented favorably on the paper ice cream cones hanging on the door and walls. The cones on the door said, "Welcome to Mr. Cohen's Class." On the walls, I had written the name of each student on a brightly colored ice cream cone.

Everyone in the room, including me, was excited. The kids were all smiling and began making new friends right away. I overheard a few sharing stories about why they were picked over other students in their class, and they were discussing how some of the other students were upset that they were not picked to be in my class. It made me feel great to hear that.

First things first, I decided. I needed to figure out who these kids were; I needed to get to know them. I got my student list and began to go down the roster, all the while feeling like I was announcing the starting lineup for an all-star baseball game. I was that proud.

When I finished, I noticed there was one little girl who was not on my list. I went to Hilarie and she quickly figured out the situation. This girl was not on the list to switch classes, but she so badly wanted to be in my class that she had made the switch on her own. Her teacher had never even realized she had left the room. I was very flattered, but quickly sent her back to her own class.

When the kids left for the weekend, butterflies started kicking around in my stomach. I was officially a teacher and I had a lot to do. The only problem was that I didn't really know what I was supposed to do. This is common for first-year teachers; college teaches us only so much. Once we get into real-life situations, we have to make it work on our own. I knew that only time and experience would make me more comfortable, and I tried not to stress out too much.

The next week I had an open house for my class. Ours was the only class doing an open house because all the other classes had held theirs just after the school year started. This was a great chance for me to meet the parents. I talked about Tourette's, but that didn't take as long as I had expected. Apparently I had done a good job of educating the kids, and they had gone home and told their parents all about it. Several of the parents felt comfortable enough to offer to come in each week to help in the classroom, and I was strengthened by their support.

Overall, I felt the need to prove myself to everyone. I was a twenty-two-year-old guy fresh out of college, and I knew everyone was wondering if I really could teach with Tourette's. Although I stayed positive, I knew there was a hint of doubt in everyone else's mind. I intended to put that to rest as soon as possible. I made a point to be as funny and outgoing as possible and to spend as much time getting to know the teachers and staff as I did the kids.

Each grade level at Mountain View worked as a team. The teachers all worked together and shared ideas regularly. It was a wonderful, nonthreatening environment for me. That first year, I did a lot of listening. I was very interested to hear what the other teachers had done in the past, what had worked, and what had not worked. When I felt I had a good idea to share, I would share it, but I understood that I had a lot to learn and was more thankful every day that these teachers were willing to help.

My first class was an interesting combination of students. There were eleven boys and eight girls. Some of them were really rough, and I couldn't help but think about how each of these kids had ended up in my class. The other teachers had chosen which students would be transferred from their class to mine. Some gave me the children they didn't want in their classes because those particular kids would be difficult for them to teach. Other kids ended up in my class because the original teacher thought they would benefit from some positive male support. Some of the boys were a special handful. They monopolized my time, and I had to deal with a lot of academic and behavioral issues with them. I worked really hard that year to be sure I made a difference in each one of my students' lives. And I got to know some of their parents very well.

As the year went on, I gave up many planning periods and lunch hours to go into as many classes of the other grades as I could, to teach them about Tourette's. After just a month, the entire school knew why there was a teacher walking down the hallway barking. I must have done my job well, because before too long, kids of all ages would wave to me in the halls. Brothers and sisters of my own students would stop by and say hi in the morning before classes, or in the afternoon before they went to their buses.

The teachers got to know me better as we attended in-service workshops at other schools or just hung out together after school. As often as possible, I got up in front of groups of teachers and explained Tourette's and answered all their questions. It was nice to know I had a family of teachers at Mountain View—and in surrounding schools—after only a few months.

It was nice, also, to finally be able to tell my parents that I had a job. It relieved a lot of stress for both of them, particularly my mom, who had always made it clear that her door was open should I want to go back to St. Louis. During that first year, my mom came to visit me at school, and Dad and Diane also stopped by to read to my class.

While my dad was waiting for me when he came to visit, he had a few minutes to chat with our school secretary, Nancy Bazemore. "Eventually we could hear Brad coming down the hall toward us," recalled Nancy, " because he was making noises, as he usually does. As Brad got closer and closer, and the noises got louder and louder, his dad turned to me and very dryly said, 'Hide-and-seek never was Brad's game.'"

✳   ✳   ✳

Once I finally got into the classroom, I could truly be me. My second-graders, like young children everywhere, were not caught up in how people are different, so they were unfazed by my Tourette's. As the days passed, I understood more and more that teaching was what I was born to do. I wanted school to be fun, but I also realized that since all my kids were individuals, not every activity would speak to every child.

As I taught, I used all the techniques I had learned in college, and I tried new things that I learned throughout the year. I was not afraid to try something a little different. Keeping the students' best interests in mind, I needed them to learn the curriculum, but I didn't want to be a teacher who gave out ditto sheets and had the kids do desk-work all day. Instead, I integrated the curriculum, teaching science and social studies with reading and math. We did lots of projects so the kids could participate in hands-on learning activities. My classroom was set up so that kids sat together in groups of four, which was perfect for when we needed to do things in small groups.

For example, we did a big space unit for which I had all the kids get in groups and make the various planets out of papier-mâché. I also combined music and science by playing the song "Here Comes the Sun" while we learned about space. In another unit, we learned about different natural habitats, and the kids wrote reports. When we learned about Japan, we did origami. For one unit, each student chose an animal, researched it, and then gave a speech. For most of the units, we made colorful displays on the walls of the room out of butcher paper and construction paper. I had the weekly spelling words hanging on the wall, and every day we did something with the calendar. I love pumpkins, so we had a big unit on pumpkins and did a lot of hands-on learning with the many pumpkins I had brought into the classroom. Then we cooked them to make pumpkin food items. I also read to the class every day and saved time for independent reading. When I was busy helping one student, I put on my Dr. Seuss *The Cat in the Hat* hat so that the others would know not to interrupt. Whenever possible, I made learning fun.

Mountain View Elementary is the kind of school where moms and dads are very involved, and I worked hard to earn the respect of my students' parents. I knew my kids' learning styles inside and out, and at parent-teacher conferences I provided parents with full reports on how their child was progressing in reading and math. I worked with kids one-on-one as much as I could, and I learned how to set up my room in stations, so that some kids could work independently while I taught small groups. Everything fell into place.

"I remember the first time I saw Brad interact with his students," recalled Cindy Bergeron, the computer lab instructor at Mountain View. "I was in the lab when Brad came in with his second-graders. He seemed like all the other teachers in our school, except that he had Tourette syndrome. The moment that really sticks in my memory is when Brad wanted the students to stop working, line up, and leave the lab. I had watched other teachers yell, threaten, and flip the lights off and on to get the attention of their students. Instead, Brad called out, 'If you can hear me, do the Mickey Mouse.' Several children lined up and put their hands over their heads like Brad. Next he called out, 'If you can hear me, do the Scooby-Doo.' More children quickly got in line and began to do the twist. Soon Brad had the attention of the entire class because they wanted to hear what he had to say. He made learning fun. Brad had accomplished his goal quickly, and without raising his voice. I knew then that Brad was different, not because he had Tourette syndrome but because he was a great teacher."

I don't know if I was a great teacher then or not, but my kids sure had fun. With my star chart and Reach for the Stars theme, the class could earn stars for good behavior in the classroom and the school. Once they earned 100 stars, the class got a celebration. The first time they reached this goal, they decided to have a sleep-out during the day under the stars, since we were learning about planets. The kids brought sleeping bags and we made s'mores. I don't know who enjoyed that day more, the kids or me.

I used a flip chart with colored cards to monitor behavior. Each child had a pocket and began the day with a yellow pocket card for good behavior. If a student misbehaved, he or she had to flip the card to another color that meant time-out. A second misbehavior and the student flipped the card to a color that meant he or she had to miss recess, and so on until the child eventually ended up in the principal's office. I tried to deal with the problem myself before it got that far, because my own trips to the principal's office were still fresh in my mind, and I knew what a negative and devastating experience that could be.

Keeping order in the classroom was really hard for me that first year. I had several children who decided to write "bad words" on the back wall of the school. Discipline aside, as a first-year teacher I was most surprised to see that these children spelled the bad words correctly, while missing simple words on their spelling tests. I had several students who were discipline problems, and I didn't know as much as the veteran teachers about how to take charge. When two students tried to light a match in the bathroom, the other teachers and Hilarie were there to help me.

Lighting a match in the bathroom was not acceptable behavior by any means. Together, Hilarie, the other teachers, and I decided on firmness, but also a program of extra attention and strong praise for the smallest successes. The plan worked, and I am happy to say that a few years later both children were doing well. To me, that is what teaching is about. I happened to be in those children's lives at a critical time and for some reason recognized it as such. Had the situation been handled poorly, those kids could have ended up as arsonists incarcerated in juvenile detention. Instead, they found positive alternatives and they are turning into productive young citizens.

Late in the year, another of my toughest kids gave me a poem, and attached to it was a penny with the shape of an apple cut out of it. That poem is one of my most treasured possessions, because it means that in some way I touched that child's life. I never look at it without thinking of that kid, and I'm so very proud that I could make a difference.

After the match incident, I turned often to another second grade teacher, Susan Scott, for help in deciding how to deal with problems in my classroom. Susan became a mentor to me as she helped me with curriculum and routine problems.

And there were certainly many problems, both before and after I was seeking advice from Susan. We had a fire drill my first day of school, and I took my class out the wrong door. If that wasn't embarrassing enough, the entire school had to do the drill again because my class had messed up in front of the fire marshal. As the year went on, more happened. I ran out of pencils the first month; then I sent home a newsletter with some major misspellings; once, I forgot to save some permission slips for a field trip, so the morning of the outing I had to call each parent to confirm that we had permission to take their child to a museum.

In spite of glitches like these, my daily routine rarely varied and I thrived on the structure of my days. I'd arrive at school a little early and get situated before the kids came. We did reading, writing, and math in the morning, social studies and science in the afternoon. In between were lunch and recess. Some of the teachers sent out for their lunch, but I ate the school lunch. Early on, I got in good with the lunchroom server. She quickly learned what I liked and what I didn't like, and made sure that I always had a big helping of vegetables to go with the two chocolate-chip cookies I'd take consistently. I have to say that the food at Mountain View really was very good—certainly better than the fast food I was eating for dinner.

In the spring of that year I brought out the bubble. This was a huge piece of plastic attached to a fan. The fan blew into the plastic, forming a tentlike bubble, and four or five kids at a time could go inside where it was quiet and cool to read or study. The kids loved this ten-foot-wide bubble, and it became one of my trademarks.

I also took lots of pictures of my first class. A teacher doesn't get a second chance for a first class, so I wanted to have plenty of photos to remember everything we did. One day while I was trying to take a class picture, the kids wanted everyone to make a funny face. I just could not get them to smile for my nice photo, and I realized I would never have a nice photo of my class if I let them make funny faces every time. So I told them that every time we took a class picture, I would take two pictures. For the first one, everyone would smile. For the second one, everyone would make the goofiest face possible. This strategy yielded some hilarious results.

As the year progressed, I worked with the children who struggled in reading, spent a lot of time with the kids who couldn't write well, redirected bad behavior, and challenged the kids who needed to be challenged. I went to Susan, my mentor teacher, and told her I was having a good first-year experience, but I often felt like I was not really sure if what I was teaching was good enough. In reply, she gave me a sign that I still have on my desk. It reads: "IF YOU WANT TO FEEL SECURE, DO WHAT YOU ALREADY KNOW HOW TO DO. IF YOU WANT TO BE A TRUE PROFESSIONAL AND CONTINUE TO GROW . . . GO TO THE CUT-TING EDGE OF YOUR COMPETENCE, WHICH MEANS A TEMPORARY LOSS OF SECURITY. SO WHENEVER YOU DON'T QUITE KNOW WHAT YOU'RE DOING, KNOW YOU'RE GROWING." This quote from renowned educator Madeline Hunter still guides me as I plan my days.

12

Going to the Cutting Edge

One day in early March 1997, when I was about six months into the job, Hilarie pulled me into her office and told me she wanted to nominate me for an award. The Sallie Mae First Class Teacher of the Year Award was given in every state and Washington, D.C., to their best first-year teachers. First, each school in each county decides if there is anyone from their school they'd like to nominate. Then each county chooses a winning teacher from its individual schools. Then each state chooses a winning teacher out of all its county winners. Mountain View wanted to put my name in for their school.

I was very flattered, but after taking the application home and reading it, I really didn't think the award was for me. The next day I walked into Hilarie's office and said, "I think I'd like to decline the nomination right now."

"Why would you do that?" she asked, a very puzzled look on her face.

I tried to explain why I didn't think I deserved the nomination. I knew I did a good job as a second grade teacher, but I knew there were many areas in which I needed to improve, such as in learning how to maintain discipline in the classroom. I knew I could do better.

Hilarie explained to me that she thought I had an excellent chance to win the award because I had done so many good things for so many kids and faculty members. She reminded me of the special things I did and asked me to reconsider. Once again I said, "Thanks, but no thanks."

But as I was leaving her office, I decided to think about it that evening. The application would still be on her desk in the morning.

"We get a lot of new teachers," said Hilarie a few years later, "but before I met Brad, there was never anyone I really considered exceptional—no one I ever considered nominating for this award. Brad had to leap so many hurdles and he went above and beyond with the kids each and every day. He was so confident in himself that his students became more confident in themselves. The nomination was not a difficult thing to do for Brad."

I was honored that Hilarie thought of me for this. But I really didn't think I deserved the nomination. I had won awards before, and each one felt good and well deserved, but this seemed different. I felt I did well, but was I really the best first-year teacher in that county? I didn't want to be considered if I wasn't in the playing field with the other nominees. I thought about it all night and finally realized that Hilarie—along with Jim—had given me the opportunity to teach. If she saw something in me back at the beginning of the school year, then she must see something good in this award for me. She would not have suggested that she nominate me if she didn't believe I could win. I had a great deal of trust in and respect for Hilarie, and if she thought I had a chance, who was I to say no? Okay, I decided, we'd give it a go.

The next day as soon as I got to school, I stopped by Hilarie's office. "WOOP! Let's go for it," I said.

To complete the application, there were a few things she needed to do and a few things I needed to do. One of my tasks was to write an essay describing the greatest obstacle I had faced in my first year of teaching, how I had overcome it, and the advice I could give to other beginning teachers. I chose to write about dealing with Tourette's, not because the obstacle was so great for me, but because it was so great for others. I was used to explaining Tourette's, so that was not the obstacle. The obstacle was getting people to accept me—and the time it took for that to happen. I also wrote:

> *My personal experiences have influenced my personal goal to help ANY child in need. When my administrator asked if she could nominate me for this award, I was very proud at first. But then I questioned whether I was good enough, as I felt I had so much to learn. She stated that every teacher, regardless of experience, could continue to grow, but that my personal triumphs bring something special to the classroom that is rarely seen.*
>
> *I have had countless experiences my first year and there are many things I would pass on to beginning teachers. One thing stands out more than anything else: enjoy what you do and reflect upon your teaching style so you can improve. Each*

teacher has his or her own approach, and that is what makes
each of us unique. I truly believe in following your heart. If I
had listened to all the "well-meaning" advice given to me over
the years, I would not be where I am today. Believe in yourself
and remember that you can make a difference.

After a few days everything was done, and I have to admit
that the application was impressive. Hilarie sent it off to the
Cobb County office. The county winner would be announced in
a few months.

I decided not to tell anyone about the application or the
possibility of the award just yet. I'd rather tell people after I won
the award—if I was lucky enough to win. That's just how I am
with things like this. Telling people before I win gets their hopes
up for me. I am so fortunate to have so many close friends that
I hate to disappoint them if I don't win. I've also found that the
excitement level is much higher if I tell them after I win.
Keeping this particular secret was not hard for me. Even though
I had already been chosen Mountain View Elementary First
Class Teacher of the Year, there was a lot more at stake if I won
at the county level. So I waited it out.

※　※　※

In late April, Mary Ellen Hopkins, who was the parent of
a child in our school and worked for the *Atlanta Journal-
Constitution,* asked if she could do a story on me. The first week
in May was National Teacher Appreciation Week, and she
thought an article about me would be timely. At first I wasn't big
on the idea because experience had shown me that people in the
media can twist things you say, and that causes trouble. But she

stopped by my classroom to talk, and I developed a small degree of trust. The angle she wanted to hit was an approach I felt comfortable with. She wanted to focus on the fact that my Tourette's was teaching the students in my class more than just reading and writing—they were also learning to accept different kinds of people. I felt even better about it when she agreed to let me read the story for accuracy before it was published.

So we did the interview, and a photographer visited my class. When Mary read the finished story to me over the phone, she told me she was not going to read me the quotes from the kids, parents, or administrators. She said she wanted me to have some level of surprise when I read the article when it came out in the paper. I was curious but said that was fine.

My class was so excited when the article came out on May 1. I made sure to get up extra early that day so I could go around to the stores and buy as many copies as I could. I wanted to be sure each child in the class got his or her own copy because my students were as much a part of my success as I was.

The title of the article said it all: "He's a Walking Role Model." That got the attention of many people, including me! I especially liked it because the focus was less on Tourette's than on my doing a good job teaching children. I was particularly happy about the fact that Mountain View got so much credit. Twenty-four other administrators hadn't wanted me to teach at their school, but I had persevered and found a school that was not only willing to take a chance on me but was willing to make me a success.

"I had a friend who was a principal at a school in another county, and she lived across the street from me," recalled Hilarie.

"One evening just after we hired Brad, we were out walking and she said she'd heard there was a young guy who wanted to be a teacher who was going around asking for a job . . . and he was barking. She said she thought a guy like that must be nuts to think he could be a teacher. I told my friend that I'd just hired that guy and that she was nuts not to. I was disappointed that she never took time to meet Brad before she dismissed him as some nut. Now he was our school's first-year Teacher of the Year and was featured in this article. I was really hoping that my friend was reading the paper that day."

Hilarie also recalled a computer course all the teachers had taken.

"We were outside the room signing in, and Brad was in the hallway, barking like he does," she said. "One of the teachers from another school remarked snidely that someone must have brought their dog. 'How dare you,' I snapped back. 'That's one of my teachers.' And I went on to explain Tourette's to that individual. I think it shows that even though we who are around Brad every day forget about the Tourette's, we sometimes forget that he has to put up with this kind of thing every day, yet he still retains a very positive attitude. That, to me, is impressive."

✳   ✳   ✳

In early June we had a staff meeting after school. This was a normal event; the administrators would go over information about the end of the school year, as we had only one week left. All the teachers gathered in the media center. I was sitting to one side of the room with the other second grade teachers, as usual. But I could tell there was something different about this staff meeting. Hilarie started it by introducing a visitor from the Cobb County education office.

I had no idea who the woman was or why she was there. Even when she said one of the Mountain View staff members had been selected for a special award, I still didn't have a clue—at least not until she asked me to come to the front of the room. Then I stood up and squeezed my way through all the people, chairs, and bookshelves. Some of the teachers knew what this was all about, but others were in the dark.

The county representative explained about the Sallie Mae award and talked about the process, adding that because the Cobb County school district was so large, it nominated a teacher from the elementary, middle, and high school levels. At last she said what I had been waiting to hear: "Brad Cohen has been selected as Cobb County's nomination for the Sallie Mae First Class Teacher of the Year at the elementary level."

Everyone began clapping and screaming my name. I couldn't believe that I had been selected. I was truly honored to be the county's choice and will forever be indebted to Hilarie Straka for insisting that she nominate me. I was absolutely floored, overwhelmed with love and appreciation for Mountain View Elementary, for Jim and Hilarie, for the teachers, and for my students and their parents.

I soon learned that my name would go on to the state level, and in a few weeks the state committee would choose one person as the winner for the entire state of Georgia. Knowing that I was actually in the running was mind-boggling. All I could do was enjoy the moment and celebrate with my fellow teachers. They were so excited for me that it got me even more wound up. All I could think about was how far I had traveled and all the obstacles I had had to overcome in order to be here on this day. I remembered people thinking I was possessed by the devil; and I thought of the many teachers who had sent me to the principal's office, the kids who had mocked me and beaten me up, and the restaurants and theaters I'd been kicked out of. Mountain View Elementary had had the guts to take a chance on me, and it was reaping the benefits. I couldn't have been happier—for the school or for me.

*   *   *

Winning the Cobb County award was awesome, too, on behalf of everyone with Tourette's, because so many of us are still not able to find any measure of success. Just after I had begun teaching, I attended a national Tourette syndrome conference and had met some wonderful people who, like me, had Tourette's. Other than forming the support group in Peoria when I was in college, this was my first experience as an adult meeting others with Tourette's—and, as in Peoria, this was a far cry from the negative and depressing support group meeting I had attended as a youngster with my mom and Jeff. At that unhappy meeting, there was not one successful person with Tourette's. At this national conference, the room was filled with hundreds of successful people who also had TS.

I loved every minute of the conference. I loved learning new things about this disorder that had impacted so much of my life. As an unexpected bonus, I found it very therapeutic to talk with positive-thinking people with Tourette's. They understood me on a level no one else really could. They, too, lived with

Tourette syndrome. I could share both my positive and my negative experiences with them and they understood completely because they, too, had experienced similar things.

I soon began speaking at various TS conferences, and this sharing of my experiences opened up a whole new world for me. Through my speaking and networking, I have made many good friends. Some I keep up with on a regular basis, and others I look forward to bumping into at the next conference or event. I love catching up with them, supporting them in their ups and downs, and having that support returned, unconditionally, to me. My growing network of friends with Tourette syndrome has proven to me over and over again that you can have Tourette's and be successful in virtually any area you desire. Is it easy? Not at all—you have to continually persevere. But the rewards are great if you only dare to try.

* * *

In April of my first year of teaching, before I knew I was getting the county award, I decided to go back to school to earn my master's degree. To qualify for graduate school I had to pass the GRE—the Graduate Record Examination—a general test designed to provide graduate schools with standard measures for comparing applicants. Many programs, especially those at large state schools, establish cutoff points for GRE scores to limit the application pool, while others use GRE scores to determine how much financial support students will receive. So it was important not only that I take the test, but also that I do well.

Knowing that anxiety increases the symptoms of Tourette's, namely my tics, I had requested special testing accommodations long in advance of the day of the test. Specifically, I wanted to be tested in a separate room, for two reasons. One, so I wouldn't disturb others who were taking the test, and two, to reduce the nervousness I would feel in knowing I was disturbing others. By law, I was entitled to this accommodation, but that part of the law isn't always upheld the way it is supposed to be.

The morning of the test, I arrived only to find that I would have to take the test in the same room with everyone else. This really upset me because I knew how much I would bother the other people who were also taking the test. Because of the importance of this day, my stress set off one of the worst episodes of tics that I have ever experienced—severe neck jerks, violent facial grimaces, and tons of woops, barks, and ja . . . ja, JAs! The people administering the test totally refused to give me special accommodations, and I was unable to take the test that morning because I would distract others. This was especially bad because the GRE was given only a few times a year. If I didn't take and pass the test now, I would not get into graduate school that summer.

I was as frustrated as I have ever been. I had just spent hours trying to get the test administrators to give me a separate room for the test, and they were completely unwilling to cooperate. Finally I gave up and called my dad around mid-morning to see if he could talk to them right away.

Over the years, my dad and I had become much closer. My living in Atlanta helped, but he and I had also both worked hard to establish a better relationship than we'd had when I was a kid. I now realized that much of his distant and angry behavior back then stemmed from a huge frustration on his part—frustration with Tourette's and his inability to help, frustration with the way other people treated me, and, yes, frustration with me. Several different medical professionals also had told him that I had a "behavioral problem" and should be dealt with firmly, so his treatment of me was partly based on that advice.

But even though we had not always seen eye to eye in the past, I knew he was there for me. I knew my dad had always been there for me when I really needed him, so I asked him to help me straighten out this mess. In the meantime, I went home with tears in my eyes, totally exhausted emotionally and physically, not having taken the test.

You can imagine what I was feeling. Even though I was doing exceedingly well in my career, I was still regularly getting thrown out of places I went with my friends, and that experience was still as embarrassing as it had been when I was sixteen. And now my hopes and dreams for graduate school that summer were being shattered. It was another one of those times that Tourette syndrome got the better of me.

Around noon, I was finally told that I could take the test that afternoon in a separate room. My dad had succeeded in convincing the test administrators to follow the law. By this time, I had been wooping and barking and jerking horrendously for hours and was completely wiped out. But this would be my only chance to test for this admissions cycle. So I pulled myself together and returned to the test center, and did the best I could on the test. Sadly, I did not pass; I tested just below the score needed to get into Georgia State University.

I was angry and frustrated about the entire situation, mainly because it was all so unnecessary. My dad had had to give up part of his day, and I had gone home crying and upset, wondering how I could get into grad school. I was completely stressed out, and for what reason? Because the people administering the test were so obstinate that they refused to give me the special accommodations that I was legally entitled to. I have since taught a number of students who have special needs, and I am always attuned to the frustration their parents sometimes feel in getting the services their children require and are entitled to. It's an area in which we all must—and can—do better.

Once again, my dad stepped in to help me get into graduate school. Over the next two months, he hired a lawyer to help straighten out the situation. I was initially denied admission to GSU based on my test scores, but I appealed the decision. Eventually, the university accepted me as passed, based on my unique situation. All I knew was that I didn't want to take that test ever again. Too much stress.

That summer I was thrilled to start earning my master's degree. Imagine me in grad school—I bet some of my former school teachers would never have imagined it! I was in a great program at Georgia State. I would be with the same thirty students for fifteen months, and I was definitely the youngest person in the group, as I had taught for only a year.

Through all of this, I had been trying not to think about the state of Georgia's choice for the Sallie Mae First Class Teacher of the Year Award. If it happened, it happened, I thought. But deep down, I really wanted to win. Not just for myself, but also for everyone who had told me I couldn't teach, and for those who have had to struggle to achieve a dream.

In July, after many days and nights of trying to keep busy with other things, I received a call from Hilarie. When I heard her voice I almost didn't want to talk to her. Somehow, I just knew she had news. I took a couple of deep breaths as she was talking, and it took a minute before I realized that Hilarie was telling me that I had won. I had won! I had been voted the best first-year teacher in the whole state of Georgia and would receive my award—together with all the other First Class Teachers of the Year—in Washington, D.C., in September.

To say that I was excited is the understatement of my life! I screamed and yelled and jumped around the room, and as soon as I could stop shaking, I called my mom, my dad, and my brother. Then we all screamed and yelled with excitement over the phone. Then I had to call all my friends and some of the teachers I worked with. It certainly was hard to focus on grad school for a few days.

As soon as I could catch my breath, I thought back to my seventh grade math teacher who had made me sit facing a wall in another teacher's room. I thought of all the principals who wouldn't hire me, and of all the times people had told me I would never amount to anything. I always knew I could be a good teacher. Now a lot of other people thought so, too.

Winning that award was definitely the biggest highlight of my life so far. As with the other awards, the people around me were very excited about this wonderfully good news. This time, the congratulations and celebrations went on and on and kept getting better and better. It felt especially good after the recent experience I had had with the GRE. Tourette's might win some-times, but most of the time I still had the upper hand.

* * *

As school started up again and I got ready for my second year in the classroom, I knew a lot of things would be different. First, I had an entire year of experience under my belt. Second, I would be starting at the beginning of the school year, not three weeks into it. Third, not only would I be teaching, I would also be taking graduate classes in the afternoons, so I was going to be very busy. Fourth, and best of all, returning to Mountain View was exciting because I knew so many people. My confidence level was high and I had a lot of new ideas I wanted to try.

I also had the award—Georgia's First Class Teacher of the Year. I still could not quite believe that I had won. Me! The downside was that all eyes would now be on me. The pressure was on. Normally, the expectations others put on me just made me have higher expectations for myself. Even though I didn't always fulfill all the expectations, I was hard on myself about doing quality work and I tried my best. I had learned a long time ago that a person's reputation goes a long way, and it should be something you feel good about. But now I was afraid that I would not be able to come close to fulfilling everyone's high expectations of me. New teachers looked at me differently than teachers who had known me for a year. And the new students and their parents were all excited to have me as a teacher because I was the Teacher of the Year for the whole state. In addition to all that, our school was piloting an inclusion pro-gram for children with autism and volunteered me to have some of the children in my class. I hoped I could be everything every-one expected me to be. I knew I'd do my best.

In September, the *Marietta Daily Journal* wanted to do a story on me winning the award and traveling to Washington, D.C. Once again I was skeptical, but after talking to the reporter I agreed to do it. This article ran on September 25, 1997, the day I left for Washington, D.C., and the awards banquet of a lifetime.

I was allowed to bring along two other people. I had a difficult decision to make. At first, I really wanted to invite Jim Ovbey and Hilarie Straka to celebrate with me. If it hadn't been for them, I would never have won this award. But then, I knew I should bring my mom, dad, stepmom, and brother, because they had all been so integrally involved in helping to make me who I am today. But that was two people too many. So I begged the event organizers to give me two extra tickets, and eventually they did. Yes, I'm not above begging! Our family had not been together in a long time, and what better reason could we have to celebrate?

Also with the award came fifteen hundred dollars. I knew right away that I wanted to use the money for education and for my classroom. My first purchase was a video camera for my class. And my first official use of the camera was in Washington to video the exciting things we did. The students, administrators, and faculty in my school couldn't come with me, but I could bring a little of the experience back to them.

While in Washington, I met with Georgia's members of Congress, who were Max Cleland, Newt Gingrich, and Paul Coverdell. Each was very nice and gave me a few minutes of his time. I had pictures taken with each of them and they all shared their delight in my award with me.

Newt Gingrich was fairly busy, so I met him with about ten other people who were scheduled to meet him that day. We just formed a line and we each got a picture and moved on.

I sat with Max Cleland in his office for about fifteen minutes and discussed my teaching experiences and education in general. While I was there, he gave me a coffee mug and a United States flag that was folded away in a box.

I met Paul Coverdale on the Senate floor. He was busy that day trying to pass a bill that he had written. My dad and I stood outside the curtains of the Senate until he was finished speaking, and that was a thrill in itself. He didn't have more than five minutes or so, but he did give me a letter on thick cardstock that stated that he had entered me into the 105th Congressional Record. I thought that was pretty cool. Next he gave me a flag that had been flown over our nation's Capitol. Along with the flag came a certificate stating when the flag had been flown, and that it was flown in honor of me winning the award. This was not an ordinary flag; it was huge. In fact, it was the biggest flag I had ever seen. When I got back to my school and asked Jim if we could hang it up as our new school flag, he said he thought it was too big and wasn't sure the pole would be able to hold it. Instead, I folded the flag and had it and the certificate framed. I treasure them to this day. We also met with people from the Department of Education and discussed current issues, and we visited the well-known landmarks in Washington, D.C.

A huge reception for all the state-level winners took place on the last night. At the dinner, we saw a video compilation of all fifty winners and I knew I was in elite company. It was such an honor to be included. Previously, the people involved in planning the reception had asked me to choose the teacher I looked up to the most or who had influenced me the most during my school years. Sadly, I could not think of one teacher, but in a strange sort of way that made me feel good. In spite of everything, I had still done well. In school as a kid, all I wanted was what I saw every other kid getting: praise, a pat on the back, a sticker, a thumbs-up. Instead, I was either passed by or kicked out. I thought of all the people who had pointedly looked the other way in my presence, who must have wondered how I would ever succeed. But every time one of those people pushed me down or held me back, the situation just made me want to move forward even more. It was as if I got my positive energy from other people's negative energy.

I also thought of the many teachers who had mocked, punished, berated, and embarrassed me. I thought a lot about them. And then I thought about the many nonteachers who had taught me so much: my parents and my family, Steve Mathes and his incredible wife and sons, Mr. Myer, and my friends at BBYO. I was the only teacher at the gala who did not select a classroom teacher to recognize as an inspiration, but I was very fortunate that I had had many people in my life who had inspired me.

After the video presentation, each of us received an award. It was a pyramid-shaped prism of glass with a quote on the inside: *It is the supreme art of the teacher to awaken joy in creative expression and knowledge.*—Albert Einstein. It now sits in a place of honor, along with my framed flag, in my home.

It was wonderful to meet the other winners from around the United States. Some taught at the elementary level, while others taught middle or high school. About half the teachers were my age, while the other half were older. We taught at different kinds of schools in different parts of the country, but at the same time we all had a year full of first-year experiences that bonded us together.

When I went up to accept my award I felt empowered; I felt as if I were representing all the people who had ever been told that they didn't have a chance—that they weren't worthy. I felt I was representing not just people with Tourette syndrome, but everyone who had a disability, and I loved that feeling. It showed that the underdog could win. We all were worthy.

Upon my return, I couldn't wait to share my award and other goodies with Jim, Hilarie, the staff, the children, and my friends. I wished they all could have been there with me because it was their love and support that had landed me there in the first place. They had won this award as much as I had.

I still couldn't quite believe I had been honored for my talents as an elementary school teacher just a year after I had sat in so many principals' offices and heard that my Tourette's would be too distracting—that I would never be able to be a teacher. Now, I not only was a teacher, but I had been recognized as a good teacher on a state and national level. I felt very, very proud. And that was what the award really gave me—a sense of validation, of confidence, of genuine self-esteem. I realized then, more than ever before, that those wonderful feelings were what I wanted most to instill in my students. Especially the outcasts, the loners, the losers, the social freaks—because many of the disasters that waited for them in the future could be avoided altogether if enough self-esteem could be inspired within them.

As a teacher with Tourette syndrome, my first and foremost goal was—and is—to show my kids the awesome power that is created within us when we build steadily upon a worthwhile dream.

13

REMEMBERING HEATHER

THE MORE I GOT INTO TEACHING, the more I felt confident enough to bring my personality into the classroom. My students described me as a big kid, and in a way I was. My second year I brought my rabbit, Waffle, to school and let him live among my students. He was a huge hit. My second year I wore a tuxedo on meet-and-greet night. I had been raised to show respect by dressing up for important events—and the only thing more important to me than meeting my students was meeting their parents. My second year I was at ease enough on "field day" to cheer my students on like it was the Olympics. My second year I put a couch in the classroom, flanked by halogen lights, and I completely turned off the overhead lights to create a more soothing atmosphere. With Waffle, the big plastic bubble, the floor lamps, the couch, and the students' desks grouped around the room, this particular second grade classroom had a comfortable, lived-in look. One day during my second year I had the entire class dress up as elderly people for a unit I called "100 Days, 100 Years." We all dressed up like we were one hundred years old because it was the one hundredth day of school. Another time, I took the class to a Publix grocery store and got food donated so my class could make sandwiches to take to the homeless.

My first-year students will always have a special place in my memory, but each class has its own character, and the batch of second-graders I got my second year was no exception. These kids asked question after question and wanted to know everything there was to know. They were rambunctious and full of energy, and I loved them all.

Then my third year of teaching, I got "promoted" to third grade along with my second-year second grade students, so I was able to spend two consecutive years with them—and the rewards were huge. I knew them and their families so well, and got more satisfaction than ever in knowing I was helping them reach their potential and become lifelong learners.

My silly hat became my trademark. I wanted my students to bond with books and reading in a way that I never had. I wanted them to associate reading with fun and laughter. So when I read to my students, I donned my tie-dyed hat à la *The Cat in the Hat*. My kids loved it. At the same time, I was looking for the children who struggled with reading, and then I tried hard to get them the resources they needed.

One wonderful day I persuaded a trucker buddy, Darcey Owens, to come to school with her truck and let the kids get in it and honk the horn. They named her truck Big Red. We did a unit based on Darcey and her truck called "Where in the World Is Miss Owens?" and asked people to send us postcards. The students in my class actually became pen pals with Darcey, who drove all across the United States. When she was in town she would visit my class, and through those visits Darcey grew to love the kids as much as I did. The kids were thrilled when she brought them all toy minitrucks, replicas of the same model she drove. We got tons of postcards back from our little project, literally from all over the world, and we'd talk about the places the postcards came from. It was much more fun than just learning geography from a book. I told the kids that if we collected one hundred postcards by the one hundredth day of school, then I'd dance a jig on top of my desk. We collected the postcards, and I danced and watched as the children all laughed and thought it was the greatest thing in the world that their teacher was dancing on his desk.

For me, teaching was like swallowing—it came naturally. My classroom was like a miniature village, with everyone doing what they were supposed to—everyone staying busy and full of purpose. I was always on the lookout for fun lessons and themes to incorporate, but my teaching style never changed. I taught every child as if he or she were my own, and as if he or she were the only student in the class.

✳   ✳   ✳

I soon discovered that a funny thing happened when I taught—I didn't tic very much. My brain was too busy keeping up with my students. The tics come out most when I am bored or uncomfortable or stressed, and at school that just never happened.

But outside school, Tourette's continued to make sure I never forgot it was around. I had recently met a friend, Adam

Strohl, who enjoyed acting and was performing locally in the play *Oklahoma!* He invited me to see the show, but I was afraid I would disturb the audience, so I was hesitant to go. Adam insisted I come, so despite my hesitation, I did. It didn't end up well. I sat with Adam's family and a few friends. But just before the play started, the house manager came over and insisted that if I wanted to watch the play, then I had to watch from the sound booth because he felt I would distract the actors. I reluctantly went to the sound booth with a friend, as I didn't want to make a scene and embarrass Adam on his big day. Later, Adam told me he was not happy about the situation; he had already informed the actors about me, and everyone understood Tourette's and was fine with it. Then at a comedy club I went to about the same time, the comedian made me the brunt of his first joke, which I didn't appreciate at all. So going out—going to events that you might take for granted—still was and is a little iffy for me.

This is probably as good a time as any to talk about dating. In high school, most of my social life was through BBYO, and most of the boy/girl extracurricular activities were group events in which a lot of us went to a restaurant or a ball game together. So I didn't really "date" until I went to college.

How successful my dating life is depends on a lot of things—mainly, however, on how comfortable I feel. Often, that depends on how I've met my prospective date. If we have met through a mutual activity, such as supporting a social cause or attending a class, she will have more understanding of Tourette's and how it affects me, because she's already spent some time with me. If it is a spontaneous meeting at a party or through an arranged blind date, things are different. She will know I have Tourette syndrome, but probably will not realize all that that entails.

Many times, especially if we meet under the spontaneous or blind-date scenario, I don't get a second date. And that's okay. The woman has to decide what she is comfortable with, and I certainly won't be comfortable if she's not comfortable. I usually make sure the woman I'm going out with knows about Tourette syndrome. The one time I went out with a woman and didn't tell her about Tourette's we both ended up embarrassed and disappointed. After that date, once again I decided always to be up front and honest: Tourette's is part of who I am and my date needs to understand that.

A few years ago I met a woman and we went out and had a pretty good first date. For our second date, she had tickets to a show by the illusionist David Copperfield, and even though in the back of my mind I knew this could be a problem, I agreed to go. The performance was held at the Atlanta Fox Theater and the audience was very quiet when we arrived—not a great setting for someone with Tourette's. Before the show started, I discreetly found the stage manager and explained the situation. He assured me that my Tourette's would not be a problem. As I did not want to embarrass my date, I didn't tell her about my conversation with the manager.

Not too far into the show, people around us began shushing me. Then the usher showed up and asked us to leave. So much for me not embarrassing my date. I told the usher I had talked to the manager, who had said my ticcing would not be a problem. Finally, after many whispered conversations, I was told that David Copperfield said I was disturbing his concentration. We were asked to move, but because there were no other seats for us—the event was a sellout—my date and I stayed in the seats we had. Totally stressing out, I wondered how much longer it would be until David Copperfield finished and I could go home. I was thoroughly embarrassed about the whole thing, and I'm not sure my date quite knew what to make of it. We didn't go out again. That's just the way it works sometimes.

I may not love the dating process, but I do love getting to know someone on that level. I'm never upset, though, if I don't have a date lined up for the weekend. I have had such an active social life since high school that it is a rare moment when I don't have something to do with any number of friends. Would I like someone special to share my life with? Of course I would. But along with thinking that things happen for a reason, I believe the right woman will come along at the right time in my life.

＊　＊　＊

Even though the woman of my dreams has not yet arrived, I have been able to make one of my biggest childhood dreams a reality. Ever since I was a small child, I have wanted to play the part of a mascot. While the other kids would run to have their picture taken with Fredbird, the mascot for the St. Louis Cardinals, I used to say that I wanted to be Fredbird. You may recall that Dave, my roommate in college freshman year, was a mascot at Bradley; I always thought that was so cool.

In 2000 a friend of mine from St. Louis, Kory Burke, was interning for the entertainment side of the Atlanta Braves organization. He was complaining one night about how his mascots didn't show up on time and didn't do all that good of a job. I thought about it for a few weeks and then told him I was very interested. As much as I loved teaching, I thought being a mascot would be the coolest job in the world. I figured I would do it for the summer and make some extra money.

I knew I could do it, but I still had to convince the powers that be in the Braves organization. Kory paved the way and told his supervisor all about me. Kory and I had both been counselors in a day camp in St. Louis years before, so he knew me well. I know he had given me a glowing review, so when I walked into his supervisor's office I felt like I already had the job.

Even though I was concerned about my Tourette's, thankfully it didn't seem to be an issue in the interview. The supervisor just asked me questions about what I did. I told her about teaching and the award, and she was impressed enough to hire me for the "character staff" for Turner Field.

I took the job because I wanted to be Homer, the main mascot for the team. But that wasn't to be just yet. First, I needed to learn the ropes by spending time inside the costumes of other characters such as Magilla Gorilla, Fred Flintstone, and Yogi Bear. While in costume, I would walk around the plaza area at the stadium, wave to people, and give high fives to the kids. I guess you could say I was the pregame entertainment. I had to be there several hours before game time and I worked until the end of the fifth inning. Then, if I wanted, I could get out of my costume, kick back, and watch the rest of the game.

In many ways this was the coolest job possible, but it was also the hottest. The character staff would get so warm inside the costumes that we would work for about twenty minutes and then take a break for twenty. I sweated inside those costumes more than I had ever sweated in my life. But I didn't care. I loved what I was doing, especially when the kids came around. I had a lot of fun with them.

During breaks I took off the costume and ran for the water bottles in the break room. I always wiped off as much sweat as I could before I sat down, but some days I was just dripping wet. Sometimes I put on a dry shirt. Other days I'd think: why put on a dry shirt when it will be sopping wet in a few minutes?

The main rule about being in costume was that we were not allowed to talk because it could scare the kids, so my noises could be a problem if I was ticcing badly. But, just as when I teach, I was so active and focused inside a costume that I didn't make many noises at all. When I was in character, I always chewed gum. That helped me refocus my energy and keep active even if I was just standing there. For me, the hardest part of being a mascot was during the national anthem—I stood there and chewed gum like crazy so I wouldn't tic. I never wanted some overzealous fan to think I was disrespectful. The worst was when the Braves played a Canadian team. Then I had to keep it together through two anthems!

Anthems aside, I tried to stay as active as I could when I was in costume. That made it easier for me. If I didn't have a lot to do, I made noises; if I stayed active, I was quiet. And good mascots are active! Most of the time, my tics just sounded like extra team spirit. Looking back, being a mascot provided the best playable identity I'd had since the old "froggy" days back at Camp Sabra.

Eventually I worked my way up to Rally, one of the most popular mascots. And at the end of my first season, I finally got to be the main mascot, Homer. I felt like a star. Homer was fun because at Braves baseball games, Homer is the man! He gets to dance and run around and generally act like a nut, which I thoroughly enjoyed. Before the games, Homer gets the fans fired up at a Rockin' Rally in the plaza. I really liked that part.

As school started up my fourth year, I decided to stay on with the Braves. My managers were gracious enough to let me work whenever my schedule allowed, so I did it a few days a week. I loved telling people about my part-time job. Friends and students would come to the games and get a big kick out of taking pictures with me dressed as Homer or one of the other characters. How did they know which one I was? I told them I'd make a certain movement as a secret sign. If no one was around, I'd break the cardinal rule and whisper in their ear, "It's me —Brad."

Sometimes I'd see other people I knew, but they didn't know it was me in the costume. I'd have a great time messing with them before I told them who it was. The look on their faces was a riot.

Later in the fall I really got a big kick out of the playoff games. Talk about frenzied crowds—it was unbelievable! The noise, the energy, and the competition combined to make it an unforgettable experience.

This job was also fun because the mascot locker room was between the Braves' and the visiting team's locker rooms. Many times I saw players in the tunnels, and I'd get excited about that. Although I couldn't talk to them—again, mascot rule number one: no talking!—they could talk to me, and they frequently did. I love baseball so much that when a major-league player talks to me—for whatever reason—it is always a thrill.

I was a regular on the Braves mascot staff for four years, and I still occasionally don the Homer outfit or one of the other costumes for special events. Other than one time when a supervisor who hadn't been told about my Tourette's looked strangely at me in a meeting, Tourette syndrome was never a problem. I can't believe that being a mascot is something organizations pay people to do. I don't do it for the pay. I do it because it was a dream of mine since I was a little kid. Plus, combining two of the things I love best, baseball and kids, is wonderful. Being paid just makes it all that much better.

✳   ✳   ✳

I still loved my teaching responsibilities at Mountain View. My kids filled my cup in more ways than I could count. During my first year of teaching, I had a lively, freckle-faced student named Heather Thomas. She was vivacious and social, always chatting and laughing with her friends. Like myself at her age, she was not a great student. I could see that she tried hard, but it took her longer to grasp new concepts. I got to know Heather very well by working with her one-on-one. I helped her with reading and math by coloring and working on art projects with her. Heather and I would sit at my desk and we'd do addition and subtraction using flashcards. For spelling and writing, Heather would write, and I would listen to her share her story with me. We'd then go back and fix the spelling of words and add punctuation. Slowly but surely, she improved.

Heather's parents were divorced, but both her mother and father were very involved in her education. I set up a separate conference with each of them and made sure they both got report cards and knew everything that was going on with Heather at school.

The following year, I often saw Heather in the hallways, and she always threw her arms around me in a big Heather hug. I followed her progress in school and was thrilled to see her blossom, just as I was thrilled with the progress of all my students.

But in the fifth grade, Heather got sick. She missed school often, and I eventually heard from her teachers that she was battling cancer. Heather went through some really tough times, but she kept bouncing back. Though she returned to school each time, I could tell she was not well. I kept up with Heather's progress by checking with her younger sister, Lindsay.

Mountain View has a very cool tradition known as the Fifth Grade Walk. During the last few minutes of the last day of school, the fifth graders march around the school and say their good-byes. Their teachers and younger schoolmates line the hallways and give them high fives and big waves. Heather tried hard that spring to get well enough so that she, too, could march around the school. On the day of the walk Heather was able to participate, but only because her mother pushed her down the hall in a wheelchair. When they got to my classroom I was waiting for her. Her mother stopped the wheelchair, and Heather gave me one of her wonderful trademark hugs.

The other fifth-graders went on to middle school, but Heather was really too sick to attend regularly. At Thanksgiving time she came back to Mountain View for a pre-Thanksgiving lunch we have every year. She was eating with her sister, and I saw her as I brought my class down to lunch. I had my camera with me, and asked her mother to take a picture of us. I stooped next to her just as her mother snapped the photo. After developing the film, I sent a copy of the picture home to Heather.

I am so glad I took that picture during that Thanksgiving lunch because it was the last time I saw Heather alive. She died in January.

❋   ❋   ❋

Everyone at Mountain View knew who Heather was, and she had been well liked by all. On the day she died, one of the school counselors came to my class to let me know. The counselor wanted her past teachers to know before the announcement was made to the entire school. I was grateful for that because even though her death had been expected, I was devastated. Naturally, when the announcement was made, my students had a lot of questions about Heather and also about death and cancer. I had had a great lesson planned that day, but it was too hard for me, and for my class, to focus. So we spent over an hour talking about cancer and about Heather. I needed that discussion as much as my students did.

I wasn't sure if I wanted to go to the funeral because, as a person with Tourette's, I had not attended many funerals. My barking was sure to be prominent at a stressful time like this, and added to all the grief over the death of a child, it might make my presence too much for everyone. But there would be a wake the evening before the funeral. A few of the other teachers were going, so I decided I could honor Heather in that way, by going to the wake.

When I arrived, you can imagine all the emotions I was feeling. It was unthinkable that this friendly, energetic young girl did not have the opportunity to live out her life. It was senseless to me. I saw a lot of people there whom I knew, and there was some comfort in having familiar faces around. Many of the mourners were young friends of Heather's. As difficult as I'm sure it was for them, I was glad to see that they were there. Heather would have liked that.

I stood as discreetly as possible in the back of the room, talking quietly to a few people. On the other side of the room was Heather, lying in an open coffin. It was at that point I decided I did not want to see her. I was used to closed caskets, which are traditional in the Jewish religion, but I also didn't want to start ticcing a lot when I went up to the coffin. I thought it would disturb people and distract from the solemnity of the wake.

Eventually I saw Heather's mother and father, and both seemed genuinely pleased to see me. I was glad I could bring a smile to their faces, however brief it was. They both came over to hug me, and in the middle of an embrace, Heather's mother said something totally unexpected.

"Heather loved being in your class; you were her very favorite teacher," said Debbie Thomas as she pulled away. "Heather loved going back to school to visit you. I know she knows you are here and she knows you are thinking about her."

There was silence for a moment. Then Debbie added, "She was so special. I just don't want people to forget about her."

I consoled Debbie with the thought that her daughter was such a lively, engaging person that she made a good impression on everyone she met. "No one who ever met her could ever forget her," I said. I meant every word because Heather had truly been a special person.

At this point it was all I could do not to break down. I knew I needed to be strong. If I started to cry, so would Debbie, and the entire room would follow suit. The moment passed and Debbie asked if I had seen Heather yet.

As I was saying no, Debbie grabbed my hand and brought me over to the open casket. There was no choice but to follow. When we stopped, we stood directly in front of the casket. I was hesitant to look, but when I did, the peaceful and serene look on Heather's face made me realize that all her suffering was over.

When I left a few minutes later, I thought that as hard as it had been for me to attend the wake, it must have been a thousand times harder for Heather's parents and her family. I knew then that I had to go to the funeral the next day.

The church was completely packed with Heather's family, her friends, and her teachers from Mountain View. I also saw many of my former students whom I hadn't seen in far too long. During the ceremony, I recalled all the great memories I had of Heather. I also thought about what her mother had said the day before, that she didn't want people to forget Heather. When a person sticks something like that in my head, I think of it as a challenge. I took it very personally when her mother said she didn't want people to forget about her daughter. As the funeral ended, I knew just what to do.

I realized I didn't want people to forget Heather, either. Jim Ovbey had recently left Mountain View, so the next day I asked my new principal if I could start a Relay for Life team at school. Relay for Life is the American Cancer Society's signature event, raising funds for cancer research and honoring those who have died of or are living with cancer. I had gone to a Relay for Life event the previous year, and I thought this would be a perfect way to remember Heather. My new principal mentioned that there was a Relay for Life meeting coming up the very next week and that I could certainly organize and lead a team from Mountain View. After finding out all that was involved, I rallied the teachers at my school. Forty-five teachers committed not only to raising one hundred dollars each, but also to attending the event in May.

We developed a seventies theme of "Stayin' Alive for a Cure," and I dove into several Relay for Life fundraisers. We had an ice cream social and also an O'Charley's restaurant night, from which the school got a percentage of the money that came in from meal orders. As an extra incentive for the kids to bring their parents to O'Charley's that night, the teachers worked as the waiters and waitresses who served the students and their families. It was a lot of fun.

I had called Heather's parents and told them what I was doing, and they were thrilled and eagerly contributed in any way they could.

"Heather just adored Brad. She cried at the end of second grade because she didn't want to leave him," said Debbie Thomas. "When Heather got sick, I know it was devastating to Brad, but he jumped in and kept me going at a time when I was weak. Through all that, he has become like family. I still just can't really believe that there is someone in this world like Brad who has worked so tirelessly to keep Heather's memory alive."

In May, thousands of people came to the Relay for Life. It was a huge success and our school raised more than any other school in Cobb County: $11,500. We also received the award for the best new Relay for Life team. I was so excited about how Mountain View students, parents, and staff had come out to support this event. Heather's family was overjoyed, because it was all being done in Heather's memory.

"Relay for Life is very difficult for me—and for our family—for obvious reasons," said Heather's mother. "But along with the difficulty is the joy in knowing it is all being done for Heather, and that Brad has put his whole heart and soul into it. We appreciate him so much."

Many parents came over and thanked me for organizing the event. I appreciated their participation and simply told them that we weren't going to forget Heather. And we won't.

The next year I was on the Relay for Life steering committee for school recruitment. My job was to get more elementary schools involved, and I am pleased to say that we doubled the number of schools participating. I now chair Relay for Life for all of Cobb County and am proud that it all helps to carry on the memory of one little girl who made a difference in my life.

All the effort that I put into Relay for Life is a form of prayer that I can offer for Heather. It is a prayer of labor, of love, and of thanks for having had the chance to know Heather, and for all the joy she brought to her family and schoolmates in her all too brief stay here on earth.

14

REPRISE AND SURPRISE

AFTER I HAD BEEN IN ATLANTA for a few years, I had the opportunity to realize another of my dreams, and that was to start a Tourette Syndrome Adventure Camp, a five-day overnight experience for children with Tourette's. I would have loved to participate in this kind of camp when I was a kid, and I was just as eager to participate as an adult counselor.

The camp was held in 1999 and 2000 on the grounds of Inner Harbour, an Atlanta-area residential youth program founded in 1962. Since all the children who were going to attend had their own combination of Tourette-based symptoms, attention deficit disorder, and obsessive-compulsive behavior, it was necessary to properly educate the Inner Harbour staff. A four-hour session was given by a licensed clinical psychologist, who explained to the staff what they might see and hear, and some strategies they could use to help the children succeed.

Fourteen boys enjoyed their days at camp, and many activities were planned for a very intense schedule. Some of the activities included swimming, horseback riding, arts and crafts, nature walks, pet therapy, and sporting events. One highlight was a ropes course, as it provided a chance for the kids to work as a group to accomplish predetermined goals. Many of the kids did not know each other prior to attending camp, but activities such as the ropes course helped them bond with one another. I vividly remember how alone I felt with my Tourette's at their age, and—not that I wish Tourette's on anyone—I often wished I had a friend with Tourette's so we could talk about it.

Throughout the week, we had anger management sessions in which the children were able to discuss how they lived with Tourette syndrome and to share some strategies they used when they got angry. These sessions provided many positive and heartfelt interactions between the campers as they discussed ways to cope with their disability.

The camp was an overwhelming success, as the campers had a chance to succeed in a nonthreatening environment—an environment in which they were not looked at for their weaknesses, but rather for the unique strengths they each possessed.

The real upside to Tourette Syndrome Adventure Camp was that the kids all left with more than a camping experience. They left with the realization that there are other children who deal with the same difficulties as they do, and they left knowing that it is possible to succeed. I'd really love at some point to organize a reunion to see how these kids are doing and to renew and extend the friendships they all made at camp.

✳   ✳   ✳

Reunions come in various forms, and a different sort of reunion was on my mind one day about three years ago when I had a long-overdue conversation with my dad. I had wanted to have a serious talk with him for a while, but the timing never seemed right. As I got older I realized more and more the importance of family, and I knew I needed to make the effort to improve Dad's and my relationship. A tragedy in my mother's life encouraged me to move forward with this.

A few years earlier, my mom had remarried—to a great guy named Stanley Goldstein. Jeff and I were both grown up at this point, so we didn't give Stanley any of the problems we had given Diane when she married our dad. We were genuinely happy for Mom. She had put off all thoughts of a personal life for so many years because Jeff and I were both so out of control as kids—she was long overdue for some personal happiness. Sadly, just a year after Mom and Stanley married, he was diagnosed with pancreatic cancer. A year and a half after the wedding, Stanley died. We all had grown to love Stanley, and his death was a personal loss for each of us.

Since that time I had been thinking about the fact that life can be very fleeting. We never know what set of circumstances will bring our loved ones and us closer together, or what will drive us apart. Even though my dad and I have our differences, he is the only dad I have and I love him, so I upped my efforts to improve our relationship.

I was a little surprised when my dad agreed that our rapport needed some work. For some reason I hadn't expected that from him, but I welcomed his attitude. A few minutes into the conversation he told me that the biggest problem he had had when Jeff and I were kids was that he felt helpless. "I was so frustrated about your situation and the fact that I could not do anything about it," he said to me. "There were times when I just went home and cried, and I prayed for a way to make things better. But I would never let myself show these emotions. I wanted to be the strong father figure."

I wish now that he had shown some emotion, as that might have let me see a different side of him. I sometimes want to put my dad in my shoes for one day as an experiment and see what he thinks. I think he would better understand what I go through. I know he tries, but I think that unless people have Tourette's, it is virtually impossible for them to really know what it is like.

Later in our conversation Dad also agreed that he was, and is, hesitant to go out in public with me, but not for the reason I thought. It is not because—as I had thought when I was a kid—he is embarrassed by me. "I get mad at the other people in the room who stare and who make rude comments," my dad told me. "At times, I can even get confrontational, because it hurts me when others are rude to you."

I am really glad to say that Dad and I have taken some giant steps forward in the last few years. It doesn't matter how old a son is; he always wants his father's approval. I think I have finally achieved some of that with my dad, as witnessed by this portion of an e-mail he sent to me:

> *You have turned out to be one incredible young man. I am not sure if it is because of the Tourette's or in spite of the Tourette's, but you never do anything but amaze me with your attitude of life and love. To be honest, I am not sure if I could have gotten to where you are if I had Tourette's.*

I completely understand my dad's frustration with the way people sometimes treat me in public, because I still get kicked out of places where people congregate. It's especially embarrassing when work colleagues or friends are with me.

One day, I went to lunch at Buffalo's Café in Kennesaw, Georgia, with two colleagues from school, Susan Scott and Sandra Keeble. We hadn't been there very long before the manager came over to inform us that we would have to leave if I continued making noises. I tried to inform him that I had Tourette syndrome, but he did not listen. I pulled out an information sheet on Tourette's but he would not look at it, so I read it to him. He still insisted that since I was disrupting the other customers, I would have to leave. I tried once more to inform him that it was against the law to kick people out because of a disability and that I was covered by the ADA, but he threatened to call the police if we did not leave. The irony is that the police probably would have been more helpful to me than to him. Because I was with two colleagues, I decided that continuing to protest wasn't worth it, and we left to eat lunch elsewhere.

One BBYO friend I hooked up with after I had moved to Atlanta was Mara Peskin. She and another friend, Adam Max, and I were at a Braves game (this was prior to my working on the character staff) when the people in front of us began heckling me. Things escalated and the men in front of us asked a stadium official to move us because they said I was disturbing them. But after I explained Tourette's to the stadium employee, it was the people in front of us who were moved. Needless to say, they were not happy about it and continued their loud verbal abuse of me until they were out of range.

"After the episode," said Mara, "another person sitting near us came over and told Brad how impressed he was with how Brad had handled things and how sad it was that there were people in the world like that group. I agreed with him. I was very upset over the ignorance these people showed, and their unwillingness to listen to Brad. I think this was the first time that I realized what Brad has experienced his whole life—the stares, comments, ridicule, and constant explaining."

I told Mara not to worry and that I was actually encouraged by the situation. It showed me that for every ignorant person in the world, there are also many understanding and compassionate ones. There is hope after all.

It never gets any easier to be thrown out of a place, though. I am always embarrassed, frustrated, and hurt emotionally. Often I am mad, and doubly embarrassed, if my friends are around, even though I know they support me unconditionally. That's a feeling that never seems to pass, either. By now I'm used to the looks, the stares, and being kicked out, but my friends are not. I don't want them to experience what I've had to experience. As a matter of fact, no one should have to.

But every time I am ejected from a public place, something else happens to show me the beauty of the human spirit. So I do my best to educate everyone I come across in the hope that the next person they encounter with Tourette's will be treated with more courtesy than I was.

* * *

In addition to the kinds of places I've mentioned, there are numerous other places where Tourette's is really an issue—think musical performances and lectures, for instance. One place where silence is most golden is the inside of a movie theater. As I've mentioned, I rarely went to movies when I was a kid, and seldom do now. It is just easier to wait for movies to come out on video.

When I was still in high school—and shortly after I had constructed my ADA card—my friend Al Snyder, three other friends from high school, and I went to see the movie *Harlem Nights*. I smelled potential trouble when we got there and the theater was packed, but I felt secure with my new card that explained the rights of people with disabilities. Actually, we were on a mission that night to prove that I could and should be allowed to stay in the theater. In a way, this was my own personal Civil Rights march. We strongly suspected that I would be asked to leave the theater, and this was the first time any of my friends had offered to stand up for me publicly. I was really proud of them, and proud that they thought enough of me to take this stand. It hadn't been all that long ago that I didn't have anyone to call *friend*. So the five of us walked into that theater full of defiance and idealism.

Al remembered, "As the movie began and Brad's noises began to reverberate through the quiet theater, I recall feeling self-righteous about any pending confrontation. Of course I would stand up to any movie patron who told Brad to shut up. Of course I would fight anyone who had a problem with Brad and wanted to take the action outside. Of course I would stand up to any usher or manager who asked us to leave. After all, we had the card telling the world that they were not allowed to discriminate against Brad."

A few moments into the film, though, my friends and I faced a dilemma. This really was a no-win situation.

"I wanted to tell the world about Brad's Tourette's," Al recalled, "and explain that he can't help it and that it is unfair to be discriminated against. But I also was realizing how disruptive Brad's noises really were to a movie patron who had paid good money to see a movie. I thought how badly I would feel if someone else made noises throughout the movie, disrupting my viewing enjoyment."

As could be predicted, members of the audience repeatedly shushed me. Several people warned me that I was going to be reported to the manager. A man in front of us even turned around and threatened to shut me up himself. All the while I had said nothing—and my friends had said nothing. I felt like Rosa Parks refusing to give up her seat on an Alabama bus. Then Al jumped in and tried to explain about Tourette's to the man, but, inevitably, the manager was called and all five of us were asked to leave the theater.

I pulled out my ADA card, and my friends and I tried to explain Tourette's to the manager. I had convinced my friends that this card was my ultimate defense, that just showing it would make things all right. My friends defended me the best way they knew how, but our great stand against tyranny ultimately failed. Our attempt to rise up against our oppressors had been completely unsuccessful. The magic ADA card had not done any good, the public was still unwilling or unable to accept Tourette's, and I had still been kicked out of the theater.

"The five of us had set out to make a difference that night," Al stated. "We tried to fight, but our tactic was too drastic. We couldn't make everyone in the theater understand. Unfortunately, to this day I have never attended a movie in a crowded public movie theater with my good friend Brad Cohen."

✳   ✳   ✳

During my fifth year of teaching, I turned twenty-seven. No one said anything to me about a celebration, so I accepted that my friends were busy, and besides, turning twenty-seven wasn't a really big deal. On my own I cheerfully planned a small, quiet celebration at my favorite Mexican restaurant, a little hole-in-the-wall place called Taxco. I loved their cheap and plentiful food.

My birthday is in December and that year on a Monday, but the weekend before was highly unusual—I had no plans for Friday or Saturday night, and no plans for all day Saturday either. That just was not normal for me. Usually I had the luxury of picking and choosing among a lot of options what I wanted to do, but this weekend no one had mentioned anything and I didn't have a clue what my friends were doing. I was, however, asked to keep Sunday morning open by my friend Brian Lapidus. Brian said I should wear my St. Louis Rams jersey, because some NFL players would be signing autographs at a local shopping center that morning. He said Jeff Lapp, my roommate, would drive me, and Brian would meet us there. He had also given me a Rams media guide and said we were going to meet someone that he knew I'd love to meet. Since Brian knows what a sports fan I am, I eagerly anticipated meeting one of the Rams football players.

Jeff made himself pretty scarce over the weekend, and by Saturday afternoon I was bouncing off the walls. I called some friends, who said they were going out for dinner and if I had no plans I was welcome to join them. At dinner, everything seemed normal. After dinner, I asked if anyone wanted to stay out on the town. No one did—it seemed everyone had to get home early. I really wanted to go out—my weekend of solitude was grating on me. But, like everyone else, I went home and went to bed early.

That night some bad weather moved in and the roads got icy. I was disappointed, afraid that our Sunday morning event would be cancelled. But my fears were groundless. Brian had said to meet him there early, so by nine I was ready, dressed in my Rams regalia, media guide in hand.

Jeff drove. As we got closer to the Regal Cinema—where the sports stars were supposed to be—I noticed that there were no cars around. I thought we were too early, but then I saw someone around back sitting in a car. Little question marks began batting around in my brain.

By the time Jeff and I got out of the car, I knew for sure that something was up. I asked if I really needed the media guide, and Jeff smiled and said no. As we entered the theater and walked straight through without buying tickets, I thought that maybe Brian and Jeff were taking me to a movie. Though I rarely went to the movies, I would sometimes go early in the morning when it wouldn't be crowded.

As we walked down the theater hall, Jeff commented, "The guy we are here to meet is in theater nine."

So I thought maybe we really were here to get an autograph. But where were all the other people? Surely if sports stars were giving autographs, people would be lined up and spilling out the door. Wouldn't they? At the very last second, as Jeff opened the door to the theater, I thought, "Ohmigosh, I bet there will be people in here I know."

And sure enough, the instant I walked around the corner about forty people jumped up and yelled, "Surprise!"

Words cannot express my true astonishment. Usually I am a pretty perceptive guy, but this time they had gotten me good. All of them. I could never have been more surprised than I was. My father and stepmother were there, and so were all my friends.

I thought back to all the excuses my friends had made the night before as to why they couldn't stay out late. I thought about how people had not called me to set up weekend plans. I wondered how they could possibly have planned something big behind my back, and how they knew whom to invite—because all my closest friends were there.

My friends had arranged a private screening of *How the Grinch Stole Christmas* for my birthday, so I could enjoy the movie without fear of getting thrown out. They actually bought out the theater for my party. It was one of the most thoughtful things that had ever been done for me, and I will remember it as long as I live. For the first time since I developed Tourette syndrome I was able to watch a real movie in a real movie theater without any pressure of thinking I might be thrown out. I was so excited that I made a lot more noises than usual. But I didn't care, and neither did my friends. In fact, as the movie continued, it was hard for me to stay focused on the story line because I was so wound up and so overwhelmed by the thought and love and planning that had gone into it all.

Later, I learned how it had been accomplished. My roommate had rummaged around and found my e-mail list. Then several friends had gone through it and invited everyone they thought I would want to be there. And they were right on—they made excellent choices. That was my best birthday party ever!

15

COLORING OUTSIDE THE LINES

EARLY IN THE FALL OF 1998, just into my third year of teaching and just over two years after I had graduated, I was invited back to Bradley University to receive its Outstanding Young Alumnus Award. It was quite an honor for me, especially as Celia Johnson, my advisor at Bradley, would introduce me.

This was one of several recognitions I received in the late 1990s, early 2000s. Laura Weiss, a friend of mine from Atlanta, kindly nominated me for the Ben & Jerry's Citizen Cool Award, and I reached its semifinals for my involvement in community service. One of my students, Lindsay Hopkins, nominated me for the Atlanta Braves/BellSouth Excellence in Education Award. I was very touched by this award, and by Lindsay's letter, which she wrote as an older student:

> *My second grade teacher Mr. Cohen is my hero because he taught us that if you try hard enough, you can do anything. I'll bet you have heard a lot about disabilities like being deaf or blind, but Mr. Cohen has Tourette syndrome, which makes him make faces and make loud noises.*

Some people stare at him when he makes his noises, but it is not his fault. I remember when we went on field trips. Some people would laugh and stare at him, but he didn't let that bother him. Even at school assemblies, kids who don't know him well will tell him to be quiet. We felt bad, but Mr. Cohen never seemed to mind.

Mr. Cohen is a great teacher and everyone wants to be in his class because he is so cool. Sometimes he wears a tuxedo to school and sometimes he wears big, huge, silly hats. His class is always fun. Mr. Cohen is a huge sports fan. His favorite team is the Atlanta Braves. He likes them so much, he is one of the mascots at the Braves games.

I'm glad I got to be in Mr. Cohen's class. He taught us a lot but the main thing he taught us is to try our best and to be proud of ourselves. I'm proud of Mr. Cohen for not letting Tourette syndrome keep him from doing what he wants to do. Mr. Cohen is my hero.

Lindsay Hopkins

My real reward, of course, is to see each of my students progress and succeed. Six years after I started teaching, I received a huge reward in the form of an invitation to a former student's Bar Mitzvah. The invitation didn't come as a surprise; for years the boy's mother had been telling me to save the date. I felt a special affinity for Jacob Singer because, of all my students, he was the most like I had been as a youngster. He had a really hard time concentrating, and while he was a student in my class I had to send many notes home to his parents about his problem of constantly cutting up in class.

Even so, no matter how much Jacob acted up, I never regretted having him in my class. Jacob was silly. He was impulsive. He couldn't resist blurting out the answer without raising his hand, even though schoolwork in general didn't come naturally to him. I spent a lot of time with Jacob, one-on-one, encouraging him not to get frustrated with the math and reading that seemed to come so easily to other kids.

Jacob's mother, Teri Singer, was an involved parent and spent a lot of time at the school. One day she took a picture of Jacob and me standing side by side. When I saw the photo, I recognized what other teachers always said: Jacob and I looked like brothers. We both had brown hair and a look of mischief on our faces.

"Brad never gave up on Jacob when virtually all of his other teachers did," said Teri. "He has this ability to challenge and encourage each child on his or her own level. Brad saw something in Jacob and just kept chipping away—he would not let Jacob slip through the cracks. I joke that Brad put a life vest around Jacob when the other teachers were going to let Jacob sink, but it's true."

I taught Jacob for two years—second and third grade —and got to know his family well. He needed an extra push on almost every assignment, but if he focused, he could do the work. I didn't mind putting in the extra time with him, and when he left my classroom for fourth grade, I felt good about his chances. He had improved so much during those two years.

Later, I taught Jacob's sister, Rachel. The Singer family often invited me for dinner, but I declined, feeling the need to stay in my teacher role. I did agree to tutor Jacob when he was in middle school, though, since I knew I was a natural for the job. It takes one to know one—I knew Jacob's learning style well because it reminded me so much of my own.

The year Jacob started middle school, Teri Singer got a phone call from a newspaper reporter who was writing a story about me. The reporter asked her what, if any, lasting impression I might have made upon her children. She replied, "He taught my children that it's okay to color outside the lines."

When I read that in the newspaper, the words seemed to perfectly describe the fundamental task of educating Jacob—he was an outside-the-lines kind of kid. But when I arrived at his Bar Mitzvah, I was taken aback by my former student's progress—namely his poise and his good manners. He still had that silly streak, but he had matured enough to know when it was important to rein it in and be serious. It was great to see him, and after a huge hug we talked for almost five minutes—a long time when there are lots of people to see.

At the reception, Jacob's family had posted photos for friends and relatives to see. Everyone gathered around the display, pointing at photos of Jacob as a baby and as a little boy. I overheard several people talking about a particular photo of Jacob with one of his teachers. "He did amazing things for Jacob," said one guest. When I got close enough to the display, I immediately recognized the picture of interest—there was Jacob with his baseball cap turned backward, and I was standing next to him in the tuxedo I always wore on meet-and-greet nights. We both wore huge, mischievous grins, and I proudly realized that the teacher the people were talking about was me!

One of the most important parts of a Bar Mitzvah is the candle lighting ceremony. It usually takes place at the reception and is a tradition used to thank the ten most important people in the young man's life. Jacob described each person before he called his or her name, telling the crowd why that person had such a big influence on his life. One by one, Jacob called up his parents and other relatives to light a candle with him. Then Jacob said he wanted to bring up a person who was a huge influence on him, a man who was his hero. He explained that this person had helped him mature and learn leadership skills, and had given him confidence and self-esteem when he had none—and then he called my name. I was shocked and thrilled and totally surprised! I never in my wildest dreams thought I'd be part of this very important ceremony. I excitedly made my way to the front and Jacob and I hugged. Then we lit a candle together while the attendees applauded like crazy. That remains one of the proudest moments of my life.

"I wanted to recognize Mr. Cohen because as a teacher he pushed me to do things I didn't think I could do," said Jacob later. "He never would accept anything less than what he considered my best from me. Mr. Cohen was a major influence on me and I felt that I owed him a public acknowledgement for all that he had done for me, and one way I could do that was to recognize him at my Bar Mitzvah."

I've heard some teachers say that students like Jacob make us earn our money. I don't see it that way. For me, Jacob was and is what teaching is all about. It goes so much deeper than simply teaching kids to read and write; the real challenge is finding ways to show them how to make the best of what they have—and then convincing them that they can succeed with what they have, no matter what. Until Jacob's Bar Mitzvah, I never knew how much influence I had had on his young life. Teachers never really know all the lives they touch and in what ways. Sometimes, as with Jacob Singer, they get to find out in the most unexpected of ways.

* * *

As the days and years pass I realize how lucky I am to be a teacher. I never get tired of it—and how could I? There are always new ways to help kids learn. And there are always new and outrageous things that kids are sure to do and say. Still, I knew early on in my teaching career that I wanted to keep moving forward. So, it wasn't too long after I received my master's degree in 1998 that I began, yet again, looking ahead. As much as I enjoyed teaching, I felt a pull to a position I once never dreamed I could aspire to. I wanted to be a principal.

By this time it was making sense to me that I wanted to head an entire school, because I have always loved taking on leadership responsibilities. As a principal I could work to create an atmosphere in which *every child in the whole school* is loved and valued, treated as an individual with his or her own personality and learning style.

So I went back to Georgia State, this time to get a specialist degree in education. A specialist degree, one step above a master's degree, was the first step in moving out of the classroom and into administration. As in my graduate program, I was one of the youngest people in my class. After earning the specialist degree, in 2000, I thought about forging ahead to my doctorate, but decided to wait because I was so young. I knew I would appreciate and get more out of a doctoral program when I had a few more years of classroom experience under my belt. But the specialist degree would allow me, at some point, to move into administration.

So, with the goal of leading my own school, I started to think about leaving the comfort of the school where I'd had so much success, to try teaching at a different place. Jim Ovbey, my beloved principal, had retired. And Hilarie, my number-one fan, had been transferred to a new school. Without the friendship and support of those two, Mountain View had less of a personal hold on me, especially in light of the fact that I needed a wider variety of teaching experiences if I were ever going to become a principal.

At least the job hunting was easy this time. Principals at two elementary schools interviewed me, and each offered me a job. I chose a school called Stripling Elementary, situated in an industrial area of a different Atlanta suburb. Of course, I brought my constant companion with me to Stripling Elementary. Tourette syndrome keeps right on inviting itself to the party, anytime, day or night.

Let me tell you a little more about the condition as I experience it to this day, and how I assume I'll experience it the rest of my life. As you know, my tics come and go. We call it waxing and waning. Even now, when I'm nervous, under stress, in an uncomfortable environment, or thinking about Tourette's, I'll tic more. When I'm comfortable, concentrating on something, focused, relaxed, or sleeping I won't tic as much. But on average, I might make several noises per minute. Actually, I'd even say several in a one-second time period. Tics vary. A headshake might happen a few times a minute. (This tic has actually helped my neck muscles get stronger.) Sometimes I call it my "no" tic because if someone asks me a question and I do my head tic, my head shakes back and forth. It looks like I'm saying no. But then I answer the question with a "yes" and the person gets confused. So I call it my "no" tic.

What is it like when I need to tic? I can't stop until I do the tic the *right* way. It's weird; I must do the tic the right way or else I will do it a few times. Think of a mosquito bite. You keep scratching it until the itchy feeling has been relieved. It's the same with a tic; I do it until it feels right. It's also like a yawn or a sneeze, in that I can feel it coming and I can't stop, but it doesn't hurt—at least it doesn't when I make my noises.

Other tics, such as the neck jerks, do hurt. My muscles get sore, and sometimes I jerk so hard and so often—as I described after the worst interview of all—that my skin is rubbed raw from hitting my shirt collar. That's why it is so difficult for me to have all the buttons buttoned on a shirt. My neck twitches start up and then my neck gets irritated. I enjoy open shirts far more.

There is no doubt that the tics take an emotional toll on me. When I go to bed, it doesn't take me long to conk out. My body is physically tired from all the tics. Imagine yourself making thousands of noises and body tics all day. My friend Richard Cohn tried it once. We were on a long road trip to Memphis, and he asked why I don't read more. I told him I don't enjoy reading because it is so hard for me. I showed him what I was talking about as I told him to read one page of a book, making dog barking noises—like me—every five seconds, jerking his head every ten seconds, sniffing the paper every five seconds, and then jerking his arm out to fix his hair every twenty seconds. I told him to not only read but also comprehend what he read, and then I would give him a test. Richard said that it was virtually impossible; after just one page he was emotionally drained. When I told him to try it for the entire book, he said, "No way!"

Many times when people see me making tics, they look at me and then look at people they are with. Some people start mocking my tics—they shrug their shoulders, jerk their heads, and make noises. Other people just ignore me. Some people seem to feel bad for me; in a restaurant or a mall, they might wink at me or place their hand on my shoulder, although they don't know me at all. If they speak to me, they may change their voice, as if they are talking to a two-year-old.

Every now and then tics I have had in the past come back. When I hear others with a cough, I get a tickle in my throat and I begin coughing, reminiscent of my froggy days at Camp Sabra. When I go to the dentist, my teeth-chomping tics come back. (When I had braces on my teeth as a child, my rubber bands often broke as a result of the tic.) I also blow out of my nose when I get a cold or hear others sniffing. I don't need a tissue—and many people ask. I really don't have a cold, but I let others think I do because it makes it easier for me. I don't feel I need to explain, and sometimes I just don't want to explain, even to my friends.

When I tic, I know others see me differently than I see myself. I hate watching myself in a mirror or on video or TV, or hearing myself on tape. Others have gotten used to my strange behaviors, but I haven't gotten used to seeing myself from their perspective. I don't stare at myself in front of the mirror on a regular basis, so I really don't know what I sound or look like to others. Consequently, on the rare occasions that I see myself tic, it looks weird and makes me feel uncomfortable. I feel better about myself when I don't see the tics. It's too hard to imagine myself from both perspectives, so I've learned to stick with my inner perception of myself and not worry how others perceive me.

As I've mentioned, although I was never diagnosed, I also have tendencies toward obsessive-compulsive disorder. Of people who have Tourette's, 40 to 60 percent also have OCD. My OCD makes me extra sensitive to some stimuli. For example, I feel the tags on the backs of my shirts a lot. Bright lights also bother me—that is why I use halogen lights in my classroom. Fluorescent lights bother me because I hear them; they have a buzz that distracts me. I hear many things that others usually don't—such as air conditioners running, refrigerators humming, and clocks ticking. In some ways my OCD is useful. It made me a better student in college, and it makes me a better teacher and a better organizer for events such as Relay for Life. I want everything organized, and I often run details through my head and visualize the big picture to make sure it happens. I am an overachiever—a perfectionist—and my slight OCD patterns help me achieve my goals. I have to know what's going on at all times.

Fifty to 70 percent of people with Tourette syndrome also have attention deficit hyperactivity disorder (ADHD). But I am among the minority when it comes to that.

Many people with Tourette's do not attend college. But I did, and to me, that's big. I am one of the 50 percent of people with Tourette's who have trouble learning. Richard's experiment on our trip to Memphis shows how difficult it can be for me to study. That's why my college and graduate degrees mean so much to me. Because of Tourette syndrome, I had to work much harder than most people to achieve them.

I appreciate my current position at Stripling Elementary, where I am the technology lab instructor, for the same reason: I know how hard I worked to get here. My job at Stripling is to figure out creative ways to teach reading, math, and other subjects using computers and technology. Stripling is different from Mountain View. Many of the kids live in apartment complexes instead of stand-alone houses, and they move often. I won't see many children go all the way through Stripling the way I did at Mountain View. Many students here come from homes in which English is not spoken as a first language, so these children's parents are less able to volunteer in the classroom or help with schoolwork. Many parents work and can't get away to come to conferences. The deck is not stacked in our favor here.

But kids are kids, and I know I can apply my teaching philosophies at Stripling as well as anywhere else. Like me, many of these kids have experienced ignorance and rejection, so I have something to teach them beyond reading and math. I want to teach them how to take the negative words and actions others inflict on them and make something positive grow from their experiences.

For that reason, I have created what I hope is a fun learning environment in my classroom. One of the first things kids see when they enter my room is a sign that says, "IT's OK TO BE DIFFERENT." My classroom consists of twenty-eight computer workstations, so I call my room the "Disk-O Lab" and I regularly play disco music when the students are doing their work. It's a lot of fun to see the kids tapping their toes or wiggling their bodies to the music as they work. The overhead lights are usually off. A window lets in plenty of light, and that, plus the light from the monitors and a few small lamps, provides a great working environment. From the ceiling, I also hung a lot of old CDs that catch the light and slowly spin with the air currents in the room. I had to leave a beloved rocking chair at Mountain View, so I bought a new one for my new school, and a friend volunteered to paint it with a wild mix of colors, stars, and other shapes. The kids love it. And, of course, I often still wear hats from my eclectic collection.

The real challenge to me now is that I teach kindergarten through fifth grade, and I have each group of kids every day for forty-five minutes for thirteen days, twice a year. It's hard to learn who all the students are in that short time, but my other activities help me with that. I work with the student council, which gives me a great opportunity to instill leadership abilities in these students. And, since I teach virtually every child in the school, all the students know me and often approach me in the lunchroom or in the hallway to tell me the important—and the little—events in their lives. Sometimes I'll have eight or ten kids hanging on me or following me as I make my way down the hall.

I tie my lessons in with the curriculum of their regular classes. If the kids are studying explorers, we'll make a timeline of important explorers and when they made their discoveries. During the Summer Olympics in Greece in 2004, each student did a computer chart on history and events pertaining to the Olympics. I encourage the kids to add art and other elements to their work to make it "theirs." In a computer lab, it is easy to motivate students by letting them play educational computer games if they finish their assigned work early. What kid doesn't like computer games?

Twice, I've had the honor of being nominated as one of three outstanding Teachers of the Year for my school. These nominations are not, obviously, for a first-year teacher, but include every teacher in the school. It is a benchmark for me to be nominated, as it tells me that the other teachers and the administration think I am doing a good job. And that's what it is all about: doing a good job of educating our children.

✳ ✳ ✳

Contrary to the belief of the twenty-four principals who would not hire me, Tourette syndrome is not a problem in my classroom or in my work. The kids don't even blink when I insert a series of woops in the middle of a lesson, or when I scoot up to them on my rolling chair in the middle of some facial grimaces to check their work. Instead, because my Tourette's is so relentlessly persistent, it keeps me determined to focus on the task of showing my students that the impossible can be truly possible.

I look at life this way: I choose the road I'll take. Do I choose the straight road, that is, the easy road? Or do I choose the curvy road? I have decided to take the curvy road. I feel successful when life is more adventurous and challenging. For me, the curvy road builds character. It's my path and I don't regret it for an instant. We all have our individual circumstances. We all play the hand we are dealt, and we all choose how we'll live.

I hope that reading about my path has inspired you to seek some curves in your own road. I hope you'll find time to learn about your own circumstances—whatever they may be—and educate others about them. And I wish with all my heart that you will find time to look to our youth. They are our future. They are wonderful, loving people, and they need our encouragement. Just think what a fantastic place this world would be if every child reached his or her fullest potential. You, like me, can help make that happen, one child at a time.

EPILOGUE

WITH DUE RESPECT to "nature or nurture," I believe most people turn out to be who they are largely because of experiences they encounter while growing up. Although I was often considered immature, Tourette syndrome actually forced me to mature early in some areas. I learned quickly that to survive challenges presented by society, I had to believe in myself and prove to others that I could be successful, regardless of the obstacles and inconveniences posed by Tourette's.

My experiences reaching my goals taught me that many adults don't understand Tourette's because their own experiences are so different. It is difficult for them to understand how a kid could *really* be making his or her noises and jerks *involuntarily*.

As a kid, adults pulled away from me, but since I still needed attention I turned to other children to get it. Children look at life through a different pair of lenses than adults. Children see the world and say "what if" and "I will" while adults often see the world as a frustrating mixture of "I can't" and "I don't know."

That's why at an early age I was drawn to children and their needs. I always enjoyed being around kids, even as I grew to adulthood, because I've always felt like a kid inside. And kids had no difficulty in accepting me. Even now, I find that most kids believe in me. They're able to look past Tourette's with a lot less difficulty than many adults.

Because kids see an effort from someone like me—someone who is not perfect—it's imprinted on their minds for years to come. I enjoy being an advocate for kids. Sometimes I'm able to understand aspects of a situation that other teachers may not, and can encourage colleagues who are frustrated with a student to remember why they went into teaching in the first place. Many of us are in the field because we want to help kids. The "tough" students are the ones we are here for most of all. They need us most.

I always tell children that they should never give excuses, and I have credibility with them because they see that I don't give excuses for Tourette's. One girl in my class had difficulty reading, and wanted to give up or blame it on other things. I confided to her that I, too, was a bad reader. I even confessed that I still have difficulties, because when I read, my eye-blinking and head-jerking tics start, and I lose concentration. It was an interesting concept for her to comprehend—a teacher who had trouble reading.

However, I also told her that I had to read my assignments, or I never could have graduated from college, landed a good job, or have afforded a nice home. Even though it takes me longer to read something another person could read more easily and faster, I did what I needed to do.

Once students use problems as excuses, they find it increasingly difficult to get out of that pattern. I help kids realize their disabilities and weaknesses not to undermine them, but to encourage them to understand their own needs. At the same time, I teach kids to overcome their problems and help them bring out their own talents. I want them to show off the traits that do the most to make them who they are.

While I'll always be there to cheer kids on, they have to be the ones who actually do it. They know I didn't wait for someone to come to me and say, "Okay, Brad, you can be a teacher and this is where you can teach." They know I took the initiative and persisted until I proved to everyone—myself included—that I really could do it.

A lot has happened since the hardcover version of *Front of the Class* was released. First there was the four-page spread in *People* magazine. My class of second graders was very excited when the *People* photographers came to my school to take pictures of us. And me? I had a blast!

About that same time the television newsmagazine *Inside Edition* did a story, and between that, *People,* and appearing at many Jewish Book Festivals, I spent the next few months traveling the country doing book signings. Of course, I still had a group of seven-year-olds to teach, so it was a hectic few months.

In May 2006, I was fortunate enough to appear on *Oprah.* Was this about the most exciting day of my life? I'll let you guess! My family and my former assistant principal Hilarie Straka came along with me to share this wonderful day. Before the show, Oprah's producers came to Atlanta to interview my class, and also to talk to my former principal, Jim Ovbey. Oprah was kind and gracious and made me feel right at home, and I treasure a photo I have of the two of us.

On the very same day the *Oprah* segment aired, the publisher of the hardcover version of the book, along with my coauthor, Lisa Wysocky, and literary agent, Sharlene Martin, were in

New York picking up some very special awards. I am so proud that in May 2006, *Front of the Class* won the Best Education Book award at both the Independent Publisher (IPPY) Awards and the *ForeWord* Magazine Book Awards. The validation these awards give to my story means the world to me.

You'd think that life couldn't get much more exciting, but it can, and did. About the time my coauthor and I sat down to write *Front of the Class*, I began dating an incredible girl named Nancy Lazarus. She was with me during the *People* and *Inside Edition* shoots, and went to many of the speaking engagements and book signings with me. She even sat in the front row of the *Oprah* audience and cheered me on. Her smiling face and kind words have given me a lot of encouragement and I am so proud to say that in June 2006, Nancy Lazarus became Nancy Cohen. I proposed to her on a hot air balloon overlooking Napa Valley vineyards and we were married in Charleston, South Carolina. Married life is every bit as wonderful as I had imagined it would be and I am very honored that I am sharing this experience with Nancy. With marriage came two of my favorite cats, Alex and Oscar, who walk all over me while I sleep.

During one of my speaking presentations, I had the privilege of meeting Tim Shriver. Tim is the son of Eunice Shriver, who founded the Special Olympics, and he is now chairman of the board of that organization. With Tim's help, *Front of the Class* was sold to Hallmark Hall of Fame to become a television movie that aired on CBS in December 2008. I can't tell you the feeling you get when a movie is made about your life! A combination of thrilling, nervous, joy, validation, and unlimited excitement is about as close as I can get.

Professionally, I have moved out of the classroom and toward my goal of becoming an administrator. I now teach the teachers in my school district. And while I miss the day-to-day contact with the kids, I know this is a temporary loss as I am on a path that will hopefully put me in an administrative position at a school. I just hope that me having Tourette's doesn't get in the way of my goal.

You know, after having virtually no friends in middle school, I have been blessed now to have hundreds of people I can honestly call "friend." Nancy and I have active social lives and our list of friends grows with each passing day.

As for my family, my mom is still my biggest supporter (she calls me every day). She still lives in St. Louis and enjoys walking and traveling. A few years ago we took a trip to Alaska—just the two of us—and we had a wonderful time. Dad and Diane live in Atlanta. Dad owns a building company, and Diane is the assistant general manager at a Saks Fifth Avenue. My relationship with my dad continues to grow in the right direction. My brother Jeff is in Milwaukee, Wisconsin, with his wife, Hillary, and they now have two great kids. Sasha loves to dress up like a princess and Jonah loves to eat. Jeff is the vice president of Web development and operations for campusbooks.com and Hillary has become a radiologist. I definitely don't see them nearly often enough. Dodo, my beloved grandmother, passed away a few years after I moved to Atlanta, and I still miss her each and every day. I am so glad she got to see me as a successful teacher before she died because she was one of the very few who was there for me from the beginning.

My big brother Steve Mathes, his wife Julie, and younger

son Joey also are in St. Louis, and their older son Andy lives in Atlanta. Andy and I get together sometimes and go to sporting events. Steve continues to be involved in real estate.

My junior and senior high school principal, Mr. Myer, just retired as superintendent of Parkway School District. Hilarie Straka continues as an assistant principal at a Cobb County school, and Jim Ovbey is retired. He stays busy keeping beehives and bottling the honey they produce. My mentor, Susan Scott, moved to Northern Georgia and—fortunately for the kids there—still teaches.

My earlier friends have spread across the country. My BBYO pal Al Snyder married a woman named Sharon and lives in St. Louis. He has one child, Ryan. Jordan Hirschfield still lives in Atlanta with his wife, Jodi, and their two kids, Noah and Emmy. Bob Steinback is back in St. Louis. Jeff Lapp married a woman named Mara, and they have one child, Elliot. He works for Morgan Stanley. And Brian Lapidus and his wife, Rebecca, have one child, Jacob. Brian works for the Atlanta Braves.

Looking back, life so far has been great. I have no way of knowing what challenges and opportunities lie ahead. However, I can now see how very far I have come. I can only hope I will progress at least as far—if not further—in the next chapter of my life.

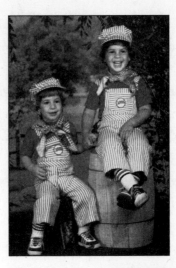

Jeff and I pose for an early studio portrait.

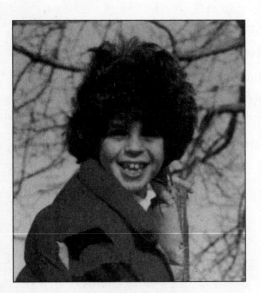

Here I am with my trademark Afro.

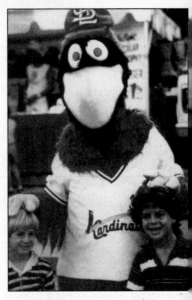

When Jeff and I met the St. Louis Cardinals mascot, Fredbird, I knew that someday I wanted to be a mascot, too.

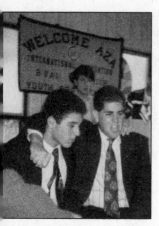

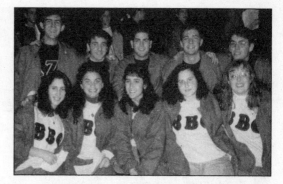

My fellow BBYO International Board members. Top L–R: Matt Blecher, AZ; Jason Porth, MI; me; Dan Wolf, CO; Scott Sternberg, OH. Bottom L–R: Meka Millstone, OH; Wendy Smith, FL; Pam Howard, FL; Alli Meyer, DE; and Becca Goldstein, NE.

Greg Litt, one of my opponents, was with me when I won a seat on the International Board of Directors for BBYO.

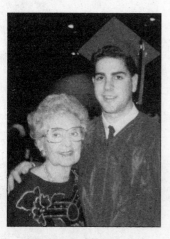

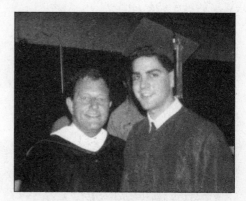

My beloved Dodo and me at my high school graduation.

My junior and senior high school principal, Bill Myer, congratulates me at my high school graduation.

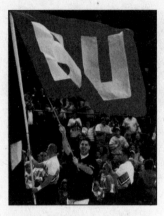

I proudly wave the flag for my chosen school, Bradley University.

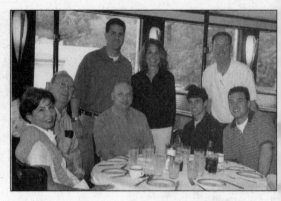

Here I am with my mom and Steve's family at his older son's college graduation. Sitting L–R: Julie Mathes, Julian Mathes, Rich'ard Optican, Joey Mathes, Andy Mathes. Standing L–R: Me, my mom, Steve Mathes.

My roommate Jordan Hirschfield and I wave the flag at the 1996 Summer Olympics in Atlanta.

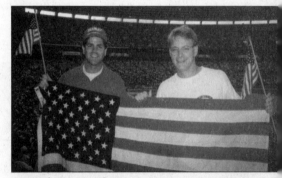

Former major-league baseball player and fellow Touretter Jim Eisenreich has always been a big inspiration to me, and I am extremely proud that he agreed to write the foreword to this book.

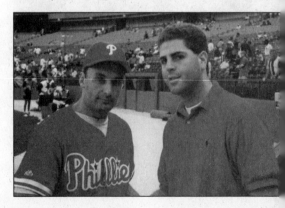

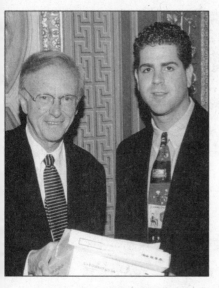

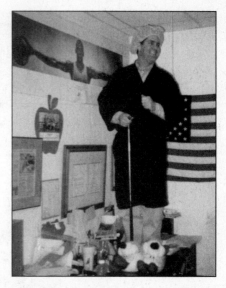

Senator Paul Coverdell and I met in Washington, D.C., when I received the Teacher of the Year award for the state of Georgia.

On the 100th day of school I dressed up like I was 100 years old (apologies to the ageism police!) and danced on top of my desk for the kids.

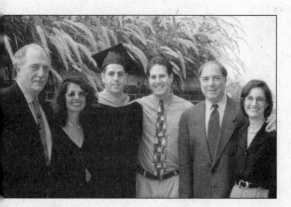

My family was right by my side when I received my master's degree. L–R: Stanley and Ellen Goldstein (stepdad and Mom); me; my brother, Jeff; Norman and Diane Cohen (Dad and stepmom).

My friends were with me to celebrate me earning my master's degree. Top L–R: Al Synder, Jordan Hirschfield, me, and Matt Mitchell. Front L–R: Jeff Cohen, Bob Steinback, Brad Burns, Tom Balk.

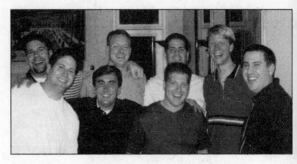

On an overnight school field trip, principal Jim Ovbey learned firsthand that I do not tic in my sleep.

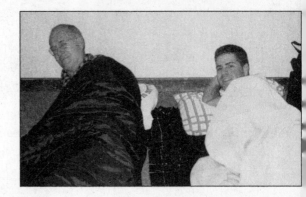

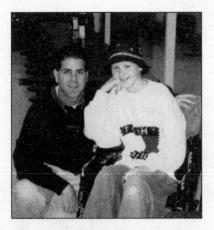

The last time I saw Heather Thomas was at a pre-Thanksgiving lunch at our school. I am so thankful I had my camera with me that day.

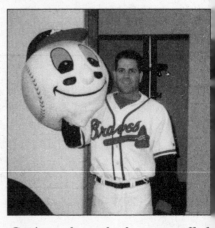

Getting to be on the character staff of the Atlanta Braves was another dream come true. Here I am as the main character, Homer.

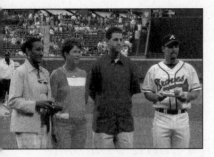

I received the Atlanta Braves/ BellSouth Excellence in Education Award at Turner Field, home of the Braves. L–R: a BellSouth representative, a fellow winner, me, and Keith Lockhart of the Braves.

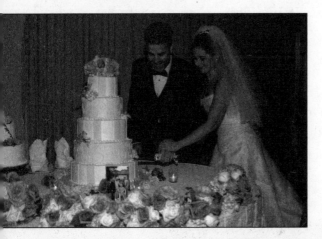

Here I am on my wedding day with the two loves of my life, Nancy, my wife, and eating cake!

Me and my wife with the Hallmark executive team. Back row L–R: Andy Gottlieb (producer), Brad Moore (president, HHOF), Peter Werner (director), Brent Shields (executive producer), Jan Parkinson (VP, HHOF). I'm honored that Hallmark produced a movie about my life in 2008.

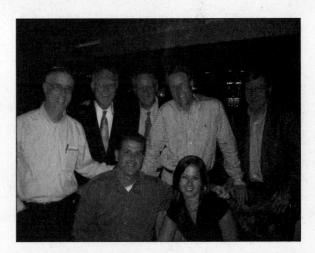

Appendix

Thoughts on Living with Tourette Syndrome and Other Disabilities

Following are some thoughts that have gotten me through tough times. Whenever life gets me down, I go back to them. I share them with you in hopes that whether or not you have Tourette's or another disability, they will help you as much as they have helped me.

Have a positive attitude.

Always think that you will succeed—failure is not an option. Think ahead so you never put yourself in a lose-lose situation. Plan your work, and then work your plan.

Success breeds success.

It's important to put yourself in successful situations so you can build confidence and self-esteem. I always tell myself that I can be successful. This helps me keep a positive attitude. Even if something occurs that keeps me from achieving a goal on my timeline, I don't give up, because I still have another chance to do it again. Find the people who are successful doing whatever it is that you want to do. Watch them, learn from them, and then do it.

You can't choose to have a disability, but you can choose to accept it.

Attitude again. It might take a while, but once you accept the fact that you have a disability, figure out how you can be successful. There always is a way. Acceptance is one of the best ways to deal with something different.

Find a simple way to explain your disability to others.

I explain Tourette's to my students by saying that there is something in my brain that causes me to make weird noises and funny faces. I ask them if there is something in their brains that makes them do something they can't control. They may respond by saying that their brain tells them to talk or walk. Then I take it a step further and ask what their brains tell their eyes to do. We then discuss how they have to blink. By this time, kids usually have the basics of Tourette syndrome down cold. Adults often need a little more time. I start by telling them simply that Tourette syndrome is a neurological disorder that causes people to make noises and twitches they cannot control.

You can actually choose to think of your disability as a friend.

Tourette's has made me who I am today and I have no desire to change that. In fact, I like to call TS my best friend. It has been with me during the good times and the bad. Just like best friends, we experience everything together, and I don't think I would know how to live life without Tourette's. On the one hand, it would be nice to get rid of it and see a movie in peace, or enjoy a meal at a restaurant without everyone looking at me, but on the other hand, TS has given me the challenges and personality that make me Brad. Having Tourette syndrome has made me the person I am today—it is part of me. I just needed to figure out how to move forward along with it. So, I decided to become a partner with Tourette's and not let it stop me from being me.

Recast your disability as an opportunity.

The worst thing to me is when other people give me pity. I don't want that and I don't need it. What I want are opportunities, and just like for everyone else, some opportunities come more easily than others. I have made the choice not to look at TS as a disability, and I don't want others to look at it as a disability. The opportunities I have been given because of TS have been plentiful. As I grew older, I realized that it was relatively easy for me to connect with children; they treated me differently than adults did. I discovered that children could be understanding and compassionate, and that they had no preconceived notions about Tourette's. Once I told them, they understood. When I was a child, I did not have the verbal skills to educate other children about Tourette's. My speeches at Camp Sabra and on the stage with Mr. Myer, along with my experiences in BBYO, helped me learn how to talk to others about Tourette's.

Making a difference in children's lives is something I take to heart. Growing up, I knew I wanted to be the teacher I never had—patient, compassionate, and willing to give every child a chance. I wanted to be there for every child when nobody else was there. Tourette syndrome has given me the vehicle to do that because I have been in the shoes of children with disabilities. Usually, I also connect easily with parents and teachers because I can share my personal experiences and help them work through their particular situations.

Be a role model.

I want my students to be not only good students but also good people. I try to be a role model for each child I work with. I want my students to look at me and say, "If Mr. Cohen can do it, then so can I." No matter what disability or weakness I may have, I try my best to lead by example. I also show my students that community is important. Doing hands-on projects with children or getting involved with different organizations is important. Pursuing education beyond high school is essential. Three of the most important things I own are my diplomas. Each of them is framed and hangs high on the wall above my desk. People can lose money, or erase an important computer program, but no one can ever take away the knowledge gained from higher education. I hope each of my students will follow in my footsteps and attend the college of his or her choice.

Make no excuses!

Making excuses is easy—so easy, in fact, that some people do it regularly. I believe that once people start making excuses, they tell themselves that doing so is okay, but it is not. If you want others to treat you as they treat everyone else, then you have to prove to them that no task is too big or difficult. Other people watch you even when you think they aren't watching. I don't want people to see me making excuses, because years down the road they will remember that. A person with a disability often starts a little behind anyway. Other people don't look at people with disabilities the same way they look at people without disabilities. As a matter of fact, people often think a person with a disability will use that disability as an excuse. You need to be the example that disproves this way of thinking.

It is okay to laugh about it.

Humor is important even in the most difficult times. I always joke that I'm not very good at playing hide-and-seek. Sometimes you have to roll with the punches, but if you take the lead and discover the ability to laugh, others will laugh with you and not at you. Laughing also shows that you are comfortable with your disability, and if you are comfortable, others around you will relax.

Advocate for yourself—be assertive.

It's important for people to be advocates for themselves. Children—particularly those with disabilities—can be taught at a young age to let people know what they need. Children should not learn to be completely dependent on their parents, because their parents can't always be there. At some point, you need to either do things yourself or ask someone to help you, so learn to be assertive to get what you need. Also, understand your rights. I knew, for example, that restaurants should not be kicking me out. Try to educate people and then fight for your rights. If you lose, be sure to follow up afterward with the right people—the management or owner. This is very important in our ongoing quest for education about our particular disabilities—so the same problems won't happen again at the same places or with the same people. You can only combat ignorance with education.

Take the initiative—educate yourself about your disability and do what's best for yourself or your loved ones.

If you have Tourette syndrome or any other disability, you must become an expert. When people ask me what TS is, I know the answers. Think about it—if you don't know, then how can you expect others to understand? Learn the facts and get them straight. Practice short speeches that you may need to give, and when speaking or educating others, learn from your mistakes. You will get better. Even though you have a disability or a weakness, you can overcome it—*I did!*

Sometimes to overcome obstacles, you can just go around them.

Don't ever allow something or someone to stand between you and your goals. If you come up against a brick wall, you don't have to go through it. Go around it. Be creative and find a way. Talk to people; bring them on board as your allies. I had lots of people who helped me. You need your supporters, too.

Know who your true friends are, and let them know that you know.

I have learned that the people who truly see something special in me are the ones who are there for me when I need them to be. They anticipate that I need them before I even ask. I have seen people want to celebrate my success with me, but I question where they were when I was struggling. When I was going through my tough times when I was younger, why were some people turning the other way and dodging me? I know who the special people are because they have been by my side when I have needed them to be there. Think about the people who are always there for you. These are your special people; these are the people who believe in you. They are the ones you should thank and express your gratitude to.

There is a story to be shared, and that story is yours.

As a teacher, I can't always treat two kids exactly the same way, because each child is different. You don't need to conform 100 percent to be the same as everyone else. What a boring world that would be! Every person is different, and it is important to find a teacher—or an employer—who is willing to allow you to be the best you can be. What works for one person may not work for the next. Be creative, and communicate to see what works.

Know your strengths and weaknesses.

I worked with a great writer to get my story into this book that has found its way into your hands. Everyone, regardless of ability or disability, has strengths and weaknesses. Know what yours are. Build on your strengths and find a way around your weaknesses. My strengths are my leadership skills, my outgoing personality, and my love for kids and for learning. My weaknesses include that I'm not a great reader, I don't cook, and I don't do well at hide-and-seek. I have found ways around these weaknesses: I listen to books on tape, I eat out a lot, and I have discovered that it is great fun to watch others play hide-and-seek.

Know how to ask for help.

Be specific. What is it exactly that you need? Be clear and concise with your request, and be sure to ask pleasantly. A smile goes a long way. And remember to thank whoever helped you.

If a teacher doesn't understand, find one who does.

A teacher could have the title Teacher of the Year and yet not be the teacher of the year for you. Whether you are younger or older when you need to learn something new, find a teacher who is willing to work with you—someone who is caring and flexible and can understand the key components of your specific disability.

Stay active.

There is a wonderful world out there. Find something you like to do and go do it. No matter what your interests, there is a club or organization or activity just for you, but you have to be the one to find it.

Use the one-chance rule.

Everyone deserves a chance. Educate the people around you; then see who is still standing beside you. I'm willing to give everyone one chance. If someone comes up and tells me to shut up or leave a restaurant, I explain that I have Tourette's and what that is. The next move is theirs. They can accept it or not. If they believe me and understand, I am satisfied, but if they continue to harass me and question the noises I make, I get a little upset. I realize that not everyone understands Tourette's or other disabilities, so I do give people the benefit of the doubt. In my experience, many people want to do the right thing; they simply made a mistake the first time.

Celebrate success like there is no tomorrow!

Have you ever watched a room full of second-graders when they are excited about something? Their entire bodies are joyful; their expressions show pure bliss. Somewhere, as we grow up, we lose that. It's not often that we accomplish a goal or have a really great day, so when it happens, celebrate with all you have. Go all out. Be silly, have fun, invite all your friends. You'll have a great time and it will motivate you to find other ways to succeed, just so you can celebrate again.

When you get knocked down, get up quickly.

Don't let life get you down. Instead, think of all the little positives in your life; focus on what you do have, not on what you don't. When life kicks your feet out from under you, it's okay to get mad and grieve and be sad. Those are natural feelings—but only for a little while. Then you have to pick yourself up and find another way around the proverbial brick wall.

Pick and choose your battles.

You can't win them all. No one can, so you have to learn which battles you are going to pick in order to win the war. Not every battle is worth your time or effort. Some battles are no-win situations. You have to learn the difference. Then when you do fight, go with everything you have. Learn, prepare, and then let them have it.

Remember the Banana Theory.

It's helpful to have a simple, clear way to explain your philosophy. This is what I tell my students: There are many types of bananas—green or yellow, long or short, curved or straight. A yellow banana can have a hard, greenish skin or a brown, spotty skin. You can't judge a banana by what you see on the outside; peel the skin away and you will see that bananas are very similar on the inside. Don't look at me just as someone who has Tourette's; get to know me better, then make your judgments.

RESOURCES

Official Site of Brad Cohen
Features additional resources for those with Tourette's.
www.frontoftheclassbook.com

Americans with Disabilities Act
Know your rights if you have any kind of disability.
www.ada.gov

Jim Eisenreich Foundation
A foundation for children with Tourette syndrome.
P.O. Box 953, Blue Springs, MO 64013
800-442-8624 (toll free)
www.tourettes.org

Life's A Twitch
Dr. B. Duncan McKinlay, Psychologist
Based on professional and personal experience, Life's A Twitch!
*offers writings, research, a documentary, songs, children's resources, a
question-and-answer forum, presentations, and other information
and encouragement for those living with TS and associated disorders.*
www.lifesatwitch.com

National Tourette Syndrome Association
A national U.S. organization for those with Tourette syndrome.
42-40 Bell Boulevard, Bayside, NY 11361
888-4TOURET (toll free) or 718-224-2999
www.tsa-usa.org

Planet Tic
An easy website to use for kids, parents, and teachers.
www.planettic.com

Tourette Spectrum Disorder Association, Inc.
A great place to find more information on the breadth and depth of Tourette syndrome.
www.tourettesyndrome.org

Tourette Syndrome Foundation of Canada
A national organization in Canada for those with Tourette syndrome.
194 Jarvis Street, #206, Toronto, Ontario M5B 2B7
800-361-3120 (toll free)
www.tourette.ca

Tourette Syndrome "Plus"
Another great resource for information on Tourette syndrome.
www.tourettesyndrome.net

INDEX